The Magic
of
Sensible Dieting

Healthy Weight Loss without
Hunger or Deprivation

BELLA TINDALE, RN

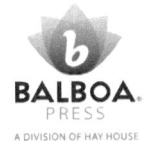

BALBOA
PRESS
A DIVISION OF HAY HOUSE

Balboa Press books may be ordered through booksellers or by contacting:

Balboa Press
A Division of Hay House
1663 Liberty Drive
Bloomington, IN 47403
www.balboapress.com.au
1 (877) 407-4847

Because of the dynamic nature of the Internet, any web addresses or
links contained in this book may have changed since publication and
may no longer be valid. The views expressed in this work are solely those
of the author and do not necessarily reflect the views of the publisher,
and the publisher hereby disclaims any responsibility for them.

The author of this book does not dispense medical advice or prescribe the
use of any technique as a form of treatment for physical, emotional, or medical
problems without the advice of a physician, either directly or indirectly. The
intent of the author is only to offer information of a general nature to help you
in your quest for emotional and spiritual well-being. In the event you use any
of the information in this book for yourself, which is your constitutional right,
the author and the publisher assume no responsibility for your actions.

Any people depicted in stock imagery provided by Thinkstock are models,
and such images are being used for illustrative purposes only.
Certain stock imagery © Thinkstock.

Printed in the United States of America.

ISBN: 978-1-4525-2738-3 (sc)
ISBN: 978-1-4525-2739-0 (e)

Balboa Press rev. date: 01/14/2015

To my daughter, Jayne Kazich.

More than a daughter, you are a best friend, an inspiration and a role model, beautiful inside and out, intelligent and compassionate. Thank you for all the times you were there for me, without expecting anything in return. I will always love you and admire you.

ACKNOWLEDGMENT

I am grateful to my husband and my children for being endlessly patient, understanding and supportive during all the time it took me to write this book. I am grateful they always believed in me and trusted that something good would come out of it in the end!

I would also like to thank my editor Jim Parsons at Oz-Edit for the wonderful job he did on my manuscript.

CONTENTS

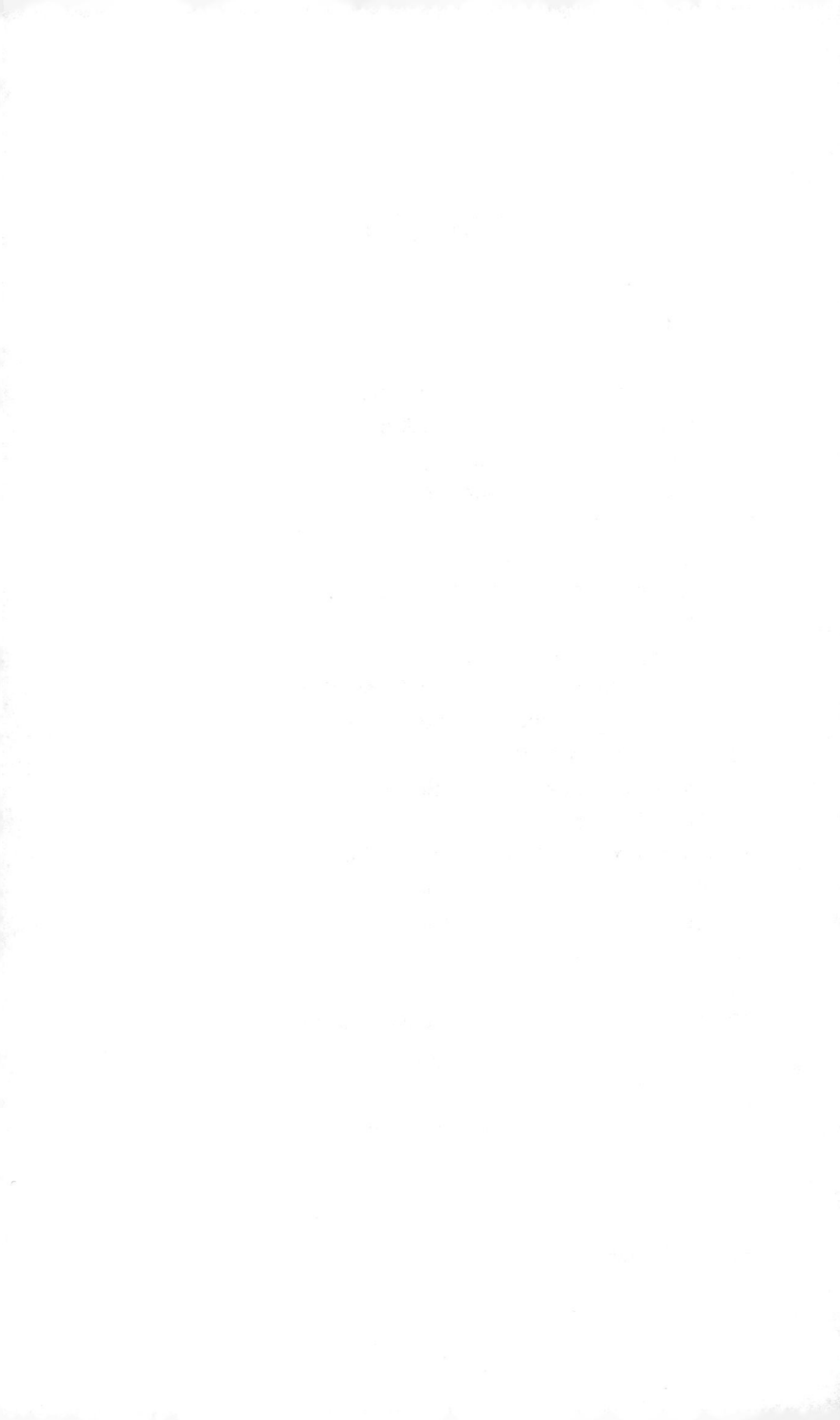

INTRODUCTION

You probably hate the word 'diet', as it sounds so much like restriction. In reality, a diet is just a way of life: it's the sum of all your habits, everything you do on a daily basis that affects your health and wellbeing. You probably got rid of some negative habits in the past, and this proves that you can do it again. If you can change your habits, you can change the way you eat and ultimately, the way you look and feel.

You are what you eat. The 'diet' I believe in will appeal to your intelligence, and, because it will make sense to you, it will work like magic. There are no complicated formulas, no strict meal plans or exercise routines, no calorie-counting, nothing that you can't or won't do. Just read this book, understand it, digest it, and you will soon start behaving differently around food. You will set in motion your personal weight loss journey, without effort and without unnecessary deprivation and suffering. You will feel better about the whole concept of dieting, as I will take your fear away – the fear that other methods have given you with their absurdly severe and authoritarian approach.

Food has a strong emotional significance, but a lot of diets overlook that aspect and solely concentrate on calories and nutritional value. This is the downfall of a lot of weight loss programs. You are left with your cravings, without knowing what to do about them. You have nowhere to turn when your willpower is exhausted (which may happen very quickly on a drastic regimen). As you read this book you will become conscious of what food does to your body and mind; you will be able to work out what food *means* to you at an emotional level. You will discover what role food plays in your life. Being aware of the psychological aspect of overeating will enable you to overcome this behaviour once and for all.

The amount of information available on dieting is overwhelming and confusing, and everyone seems to have a different opinion on what works and what doesn't. The most widespread approach to weight loss consists of a combination of a reduced caloric intake and an increase in aerobic, fat-burning exercise. It's about creating a 'calorie deficit'. The rationale behind this method is that, if you burn *more* calories than you eat, you will lose weight. If you burn 3000 calories daily but only consume 2500, your deficit will be 500 calories per day.

A daily calorie deficit of 1000 calories equates to a weight loss of about one kilogram per week. This sounds simple in theory, but it's certainly not easy to put into practice. Hunger is the main problem. The feeling of starvation is one of the worst forms of torture anyone can endure: no wonder so many people give up or don't even try to reduce their food intake. As human beings, we are genetically programmed to fear hunger and to do anything to avoid it.

Some experts tell us we should eat more protein and less carbohydrate, or even no carbohydrates at all. Some say we can eat carbs, but no fat. Others claim we can eat as much fat as we want, in combination with protein, as long as we don't eat carbs at the same time. Who can see through this maze? The advice you're getting is conflicting at its best, and you wonder who is right and who is wrong. At first you blindly believe whatever you are told, without questioning it, because it sounds like a quick fix to your weight problem, especially if it is accompanied by a pseudo-scientific explanation, such as our bodies have not adapted to grains because we're still Palaeolithic. But, after going through several cycles of dieting, losing a few kilos, then giving up and putting all the kilos back on again, you decide that you can't do it.

You blame yourself for your failure. What these experts promise may work for people who have plenty of willpower, but not for you.

Fad diets usually have catchy names and... they usually don't work. Those promising fast results can be successful in making someone else richer, but they won't succeed in making you slimmer. Deep down you know this, but, in spite of your common sense, you find yourself drawn towards those empty promises. You don't like to suffer, and you don't like to experience hunger pangs, especially over a long period of time. Somehow, you're still hoping for a miracle cure. Being overweight or obese is one of the most common afflictions, not only in developed countries, but also in emerging economies. But it is preventable, and it is treatable. There is a cure for it: losing weight!

So, let's make a start. Are you determined to achieve results? Whether you want to lose five, ten or fifty kilos, where you are right now is your starting point. From here you can formulate a short-term and a long-term goal. Reaching your short-term goal will give you the confidence to continue towards your long-term goal (please refer to my book *The Magic of Willpower*).

Everyone seems to be insecure and looking for solutions, seeking a way to obtain a slim body without feeling hungry or deprived. Time and energy are precious, and you don't want to sacrifice them, especially when you doubt that you can succeed. You don't want to waste your efforts on dubious weight loss schemes. They may be endorsed by celebrities, but this doesn't mean you'll lose anything besides your money. The more expensive a diet product or gadget, the more likely it is to be a scam. Weight loss doesn't mean cash loss.

No one can make you lose weight – only YOU can do it. You can't do it to please your spouse, doctor, work colleagues, sister, mother or child. You can only do it if it is what you *really* want. Trust yourself: you can do it, with the right tools and ideas. Discard any fear you may have. Maybe you wish you'd done things differently. Don't look at the past; look at the present and future. Make a commitment to yourself that you will let go of regret and worry, and give yourself fully to this new way of life. Don't sabotage your efforts by projecting negative, frightening outcomes about what will happen if you dare to give yourself this opportunity.

Although losing weight is one of the most difficult things to do, you probably know at least one person who has achieved this goal. Many others have failed, usually because they lack information on how it works. You too may have failed many times, but you want to keep trying, or you wouldn't be reading this.

Maybe you may think that you don't have any willpower or that you are a weak person. Maybe you're a bit discouraged after your failed attempts in the past. But you don't want to give up, and you can't resign yourself to being out of shape. You haven't lost hope, and you still believe that you *can* lose weight. The only problem is that you're not sure how to do it.

Thinking for yourself, and developing a new awareness about your emotions and your eating habits will help you get started. Feeling good will become your number one priority and you will realise that losing weight can be a joyful experience.

Obesity can cause numerous diseases, such as diabetes, coronary heart disease, arthritis and maybe even cancer. You know that your health would improve if you lost weight, but the main reason why you want to do it is to feel better about yourself, and it is certainly something you can achieve with the proper knowledge and a willingness to change your habits.

Two years after my second pregnancy, I decided to lose weight, but I couldn't find a weight loss book that made sense to me as a complete method. I would find a few bits and pieces helpful, while some ideas I read about seemed out of my reach. They seemed to require massive amounts of willpower and determination. After reading numerous diet books, I found that none of them gave me all the information required to be successful.

I was looking for easy-to-follow advice and clear guidelines to help me lose weight over a period of twelve months. Most methods were too complex, too expensive and too time consuming. There was too much planning, shopping and preparation involved; too much weighing food and counting calories, too much strenuous exercise. I wasn't willing to follow a strict eating and exercise program.

Eventually, I managed to put all the pieces of the puzzle together and ended up losing twenty kilograms within a year. People around me were more astonished than I was. The transformation was like magic, but I hadn't suffered. I hadn't followed a strict diet; I had only applied a few easy principles that I had discovered through my personal research, and it came as a surprise when friends and colleagues begged me to share my 'secret' with them.

It was the beginning of a new journey: the writing of this book. My intention was to create a simple method for those who want to lose weight once and for all, as well as for those who want to be healthy, energetic, youthful and slim while enjoying life to the fullest!

Although weight loss starts in the mind, you need to be conscious of what you eat and what it does to you. Without this knowledge, weight loss can be difficult, if not impossible. You need to consider every aspect of your lifestyle, including smoking and drinking, as well as your mental wellbeing and your outlook on life.

Everyone deserves to be a healthy weight. You will find renewed hope in these pages, as well as the tools and encouragement you need to achieve your goal.

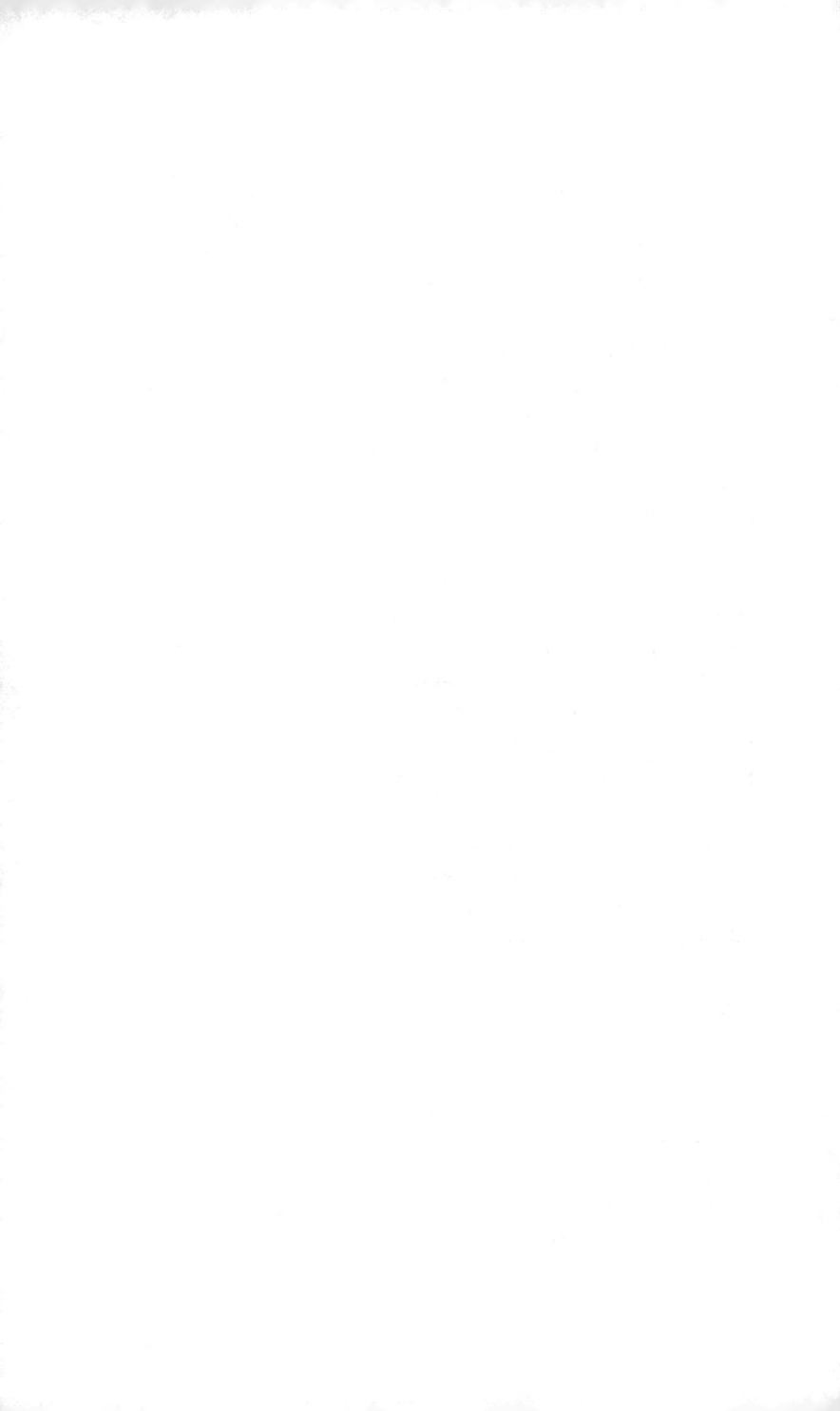

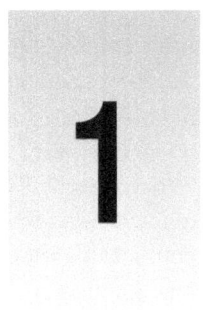

SETTING YOUR GOAL: HOW MUCH SHOULD YOU WEIGH?

Clearly determine your goal, and you will help you reach your weight loss goal easily.

Ellen, 19 years old, is 165 cm high and weighs 93 kilograms. Ellen has been overweight since her early teens. A sci-fi fanatic and video game addict, she'd spend hours locked in the solitude of her bedroom with a generous supply of chocolate biscuits, potato chips and sugary soft drinks. Her staple diet consisted of fried chicken, creamy pasta, ice-cream and cheesecake. Her mum, a sole parent, worked full-time, and hardly ever had time to cook a balanced meal. Ellen couldn't remember when she last ate fruit or vegetables, apart from microwaved frozen peas with gravy. Her mum also had a weight problem, but she'd given up doing anything about it. Ellen was a bright student but rather shy, feeling unattractive due to her body size, which made her withdraw. When she wasn't studying, she'd sit in front of an animated screen with her favourite treats.

After completing high school, Ellen decided to study nursing. Learning about anatomy and physiology has opened her eyes to the health problems caused by excess weight. She made some good friends at university, and soon became more confident within herself. Ellen decided to lose weight as she doesn't want to become another statistic. She also wants a body she can feel comfortable with. She is very motivated, and her only problem is that she doesn't know how much she should weigh. She wants to look and feel good, without being too skinny. She would like to have a target weight she can work towards.

Do you know how much you should weigh? Having a clear goal in mind is helpful, but be realistic about what you can achieve. Due to genetic differences, you may have a slim, medium or heavy build, and you were probably born that way. Accept your natural build and work with it, not against it. Going against nature will cause you to become discouraged.

An interesting strategy is to allow yourself to lose weight with an open mind, which means that whenever you reach a body size you feel comfortable with, you maintain your new weight. But even though you may feel good at a certain weight, carrying extra kilos could still be detrimental to your health. You need a certain percentage of body fat to insulate you and protect your organs, but too much of it is a hazard. Find out what your body weight should be. To remain motivated and focused, you need a clear goal: this goal is your optimum weight.

If you're a young adult who has been overweight since childhood, it can be difficult to determine your optimum weight, as you have no memories of ever being slim. But if you're middle-aged and older, the concept of optimum or ideal weight brings back memories of younger days, when you were active, full of energy – and free of the worries that literally weigh you down as adulthood progresses. It was your weight before you left school, before you got your certificate, diploma or degree… Before you started on your career path, before you got married and had children, before you were divorced…

Write down your life story, and recall your body size at different ages. Eventually, you will figure out what your optimum weight should be – by remembering your slimmer days. But if you were under twenty-five at the time, you're allowed to add five to ten kilograms to the figure you obtain, or it could be too low and unrealistic: the bodies of teenagers and young adults are not fully developed yet.

If you can't remember how much you used to weigh, because it is too long since you've been slim, or because you've been overweight since childhood, seek advice from a doctor or other health professional. Also, trust yourself and your own judgment. What may be an attainable weight for someone else might not be a realistic target for you.

What might be right for someone else might not necessarily be right for you. What are your priorities? Do you want to look a certain way, or simply be happy with the way you are? Your optimum weight is your weight loss goal, and it's up to you to determine it, with your input and the information that is available. And, according to your own expectations and needs, you can strive towards a *normal* weight or an *ideal* weight.

A normal weight should be everyone's goal, as normal weight means healthy weight. Any health professional will be able to work out what your normal weight should be, given your height and your frame – but remember that your genes play a big role as they determine your body shape. Any number can only be an estimate.

Body Mass Index (BMI) is a well-known tool used to define 'overweight' and 'obese'. You can Google it, and a BMI calculator will tell you what your current BMI is and what it should be if you want to be healthy. If you prefer to do it manually, there is a simple formula. Work out your height in metres and your weight in kilograms. Let's take Ellen as an example. She measures 165 cm (1.65 m) and right now her weight is 93 kg.

To obtain Ellen's BMI, divide her weight by her height (squared)
BMI = weight/height2
BMI = 93: 1.65 x 1.65
BMI = 93: 2.7225 = 34

What does it mean?
Below 18.5: Underweight
18.5 to 24.9: Healthy weight
25.0 to 29.9: Overweight
30 to 39.9: Obese
40 and above: Morbidly obese
The verdict: Ellen is obese.

Another example: Steve measures 190 cm (1.9 m) and weighs 87 kg.
BMI = 87: 1.9 x 1.9
BMI = 87: 3.61 = 24

Steve is a healthy weight.

Individuals with a BMI up to around 23 live longest. Once you reach your normal, healthy weight, your risk for diseases such as high cholesterol, high blood pressure, diabetes, and even cancer will be dramatically reduced. Your life expectancy and your quality of life will increase simultaneously.

Another target you may want to reach is your *ideal weight*. It is usually a bit lower than your normal weight (ideal BMIs range from

19 to 22). It reflects your ideal body shape and optimum fitness, which means something different to everyone.

If you're happy with a normal weight and the kilos won't come off any more, it could mean that you're not supposed to lose any more weight. Attempting to do so could mean going against your body and nature. But if the kilos keep coming off as you're maintaining good eating habits, there is no harm in slimming down a bit more. If it is what you wish, of course, and as long as you don't feel hungry or deprived.

To be attainable, a goal has to be within your reach. You may feel overwhelmed and discouraged by the amount of weight you need to lose. Looking at the huge task ahead of you can be too much to handle. To overcome this feeling of powerlessness when confronted with such a 'big job', you can break it up into smaller steps or *intermediate* weight loss goals.

For instance, if you need to lose fifteen kilograms, divide this figure into three. Every five kilograms you lose represents an intermediate weight loss goal. If you weigh 100 kilograms and your objective is 70, you will need to lose ten kilograms at a time. If you weigh 80 and your objective is 60, you will need to lose about seven kilograms at a time. You can divide the amount of weight you need to lose into as many intermediate goals as you wish. It is a simple, yet very effective, strategy, as it takes away your fear of being overwhelmed.

The first kilogram lost is the most important. Mark it in your calendar and celebrate it, as it will give you the incentive to continue. If you divide the task ahead into manageable stages, you will feel less likely to fail. You will feel less anxiety and stress. Make sure you set yourself an initial goal that you can easily reach, so you don't feel under too much pressure. Every time you lose some weight, you can reassess your objective and decide whether you want to stop or continue with your diet.

Being free to decide how much you would like to lose at any given time will make you feel more in control. Ordinary diets control you and make you feel powerless, but, with this method, YOU are in control, as you make all the decisions. You can lose weight and feel good at the same time, but you can only do it for yourself. No one can make you lose weight, only YOU can achieve your goal of an optimum weight – a weight you will feel comfortable with, a weight you will be able to maintain year after year, without ever having to go on a diet again.

Key Points and Strategies:

- Set yourself a clear and realistic weight loss goal
- Respect your genetic body type and don't try to go against nature
- Choose your target weight according to your needs and priorities
- Divide the task ahead into small manageable stages
- Feel free to continue losing weight or to stop at any time

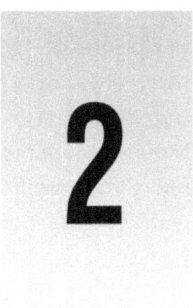

2

. . . .

LOSE WEIGHT WITHOUT MEDICATION

. . . .

Trust your natural ability to lose weight.

Eliza is 41 years old. She weighs 85 kilograms, and she would like to lose fifteen to twenty kilograms. She has tried every 'diet pill' under the sun, prescription drugs and over-the-counter products. But as soon as she loses some weight, she puts it back on within a few weeks. She is at the end of her tether.

Eliza just bought an expensive herbal remedy. She saw it advertised in a magazine while she was in her dentist's waiting room. The ad was very promising, so Eliza perceives this as her last chance. To her, it's all or nothing: if it doesn't work, nothing else will, and she'll never try to lose weight any more. Right now her self-esteem is low, and she feels like a failure. This will be her last-ditch attempt.

There is no miracle cure or magic pill to help you slim down. A product can only *promise* to make you lose weight, but in 99.9 %

of all cases, it will be an empty promise, possibly not even backed up by any proper research. A common marketing ploy is to attract potential customers with words like 'Brand new discovery or theory guarantees weight loss' or 'Fat-fighting super food will make you slim down' or 'Incredible diet secret for lasting weight loss'. What is incredible is how much it costs! If something *really* worked, everyone would already know about it and it wouldn't be a secret any more.

Losing weight is a *process.* You will begin by taking a thorough inventory of your eating behaviour, including all the little habits like putting three sugars in your coffee, or snacking mindlessly on high-calorie items in front of the television. You will replace old, ineffective eating habits with more effective ones, and unhealthy food choices with more nutritious ones. But losing weight becomes easier once you've discovered how it works for you and once it has become an integral part of your daily routine. Eventually, your diet will become a part of you, and your healthy food choices will become automatic. You won't have to struggle any more to resist temptation, as you will have released your desire for the foods that are detrimental to your waistline.

Awareness is the first step towards changing an ineffective behaviour. Once you understand how your eating habits affect your weight and your wellbeing, you will be able to adopt new principles that you can put into practice on a daily basis. Instead of being forced to follow a rigid diet plan, you will realise how important it is to have freedom of choice. Every time you are about to eat, you can choose what to eat, and how much. When it finally dawned on me that I didn't have to stuff myself, it was like a revelation to me, a kind of liberation.

Although there is no 'magic pill', there are a number of prescription drugs that can help you diminish your caloric intake by suppressing your appetite, thus reducing the amount of food you consume. It sounds tempting, as it looks like the perfect answer to your problem. But appetite suppressants such as *phentermine,* (a commonly prescribed drug which hasn't been proven to be effective long term) have severe side effects: dizziness, fainting, headache, nausea, irregular heartbeat, shaking, sweating, weakness, panic attacks, blurred vision, sleeplessness, confusion, depression, hallucinations, convulsions, loss of consciousness and even death!

To risk your life for the sake of losing a few kilos is definitely not worth it. *Addiction* is a serious concern: both psychological and physical dependence. *Resistance* or *tolerance* to the drug is also a problem, as it can cease to be effective after a few weeks or, in the best case scenario, after a few months. The body quickly gets accustomed to substances that interfere with natural processes. *Psychological dependence* is probably the most insidious and the most dangerous kind of addiction, as it often happens without you being conscious of it. You rely more and more on your medication, and you believe that it is responsible for your weight loss. All the credit goes to the drug and, as a result, you don't trust yourself any more: you need this product, this chemical crutch. You're terrified not to be able to cope without it any more.

The truth is that 'diet pills' and other drugs won't help you lose weight. The use of any drug is self-defeating and it never works in the long run, because it teaches you to rely on something external, instead of relying on your own internal resources, your own inner strength. Drugs do nothing for your self-esteem, as they don't give you a sense of achievement.

To be slim and remain that way, build your self-esteem and your sense of empowerment. Once know you can do it on your own, without drugs or other props, you'll be on the right track, and there will be no looking back. If you were to reach your weight loss goal while on medication, the victory would be short lived.

Your appetite and hunger would most likely come back with a vengeance, as soon as you stop taking the medication. This is called 'rebound hunger' and it's the worst kind of hunger. More devastating and damaging to your self-esteem, it will confirm your belief that you can't lose weight and maintain a healthy weight on your own.

No amount of money can buy you health or a nice figure, but you are constantly made to believe otherwise by the media. We are bombarded with advertisements and misleading information, stories about glamorous personalities who, with the help of fad diets, personal trainers and plastic surgery, are restored to a youthful shape and appearance.

Most people have a limited budget and don't live in Hollywood-style mansions. But even – and especially if – you don't have much money, you deserve to be healthy, regardless of your age and circumstances. Feeling and looking fit and well is a better goal than looking slim, following magazine beauty ideals. Unfortunately, being beautiful is a goal that is ingrained in us by commercial interests from an early age. You have a right to be a normal, healthy weight, and you don't need to be wealthy to achieve this. You only need your brain and your common sense. These are your most important tools, along with a strong vision and a tiny bit of determination.

To lose weight, you won't have to spend more money than you usually do. On the contrary, you will probably save some money, as the foods recommended in these pages are mostly inexpensive and easily available. The first step is to gain some insight into your eating pattern, and the *emotions* connected with it. The knowledge that *you can do it,* combined with a strong desire to become the person you *really* want to be, will help you overcome obstacles along the way.

Key Points and Strategies:

- Don't waste money on weight loss products or gadgets
- Develop confidence in your ability to lose weight
- Take an inventory of your eating behaviour
- Replace bad habits with good ones
- Be aware of what you eat and why
- Build your self-esteem to achieve long-lasting results
- Motivation works better than medication

3

THE BODY'S SETPOINT

Use the set point mechanism to lose weight consistently.

Keith, 45, is the CEO of a big organisation. He has everything going for him: a gorgeous wife, two healthy children, a big house in a sought-after neighbourhood, and a Volvo XC70. The only thing that makes him unhappy is his waistline. When he met his wife twelve years ago, Keith was slim and athletic, weighing 78 kg at 185 cm high (BMI of 22.7).

He decided to go on diet two-and-a-half months ago and has been satisfied with his results so far. He weighed 103 kilos just before he started, and now he weighs 96. However, his weight has been static for the last three weeks, even though Keith hasn't deviated from his strict diet and exercise plan. For the last three weeks, the scale hasn't moved. To his dismay, he doesn't seem to be able to lose any more weight. Keith is angry and bewildered, as he only eats low-calorie foods and goes to the gym every day. What he doesn't realise is that he has reached a *plateau*. He doesn't know that, with persistence, he will shed more kilos eventually.

Only human beings can deliberately choose to lose weight. In the past, the amount of fat you carried determined your chances of survival during periods of food shortages and famines. People were more concerned about survival than about body shape, and being overweight was often considered a status symbol and a sign of wealth. To most people, stockpiling enough food to get them through hard times was more important than worrying about ideal weight. Scarcity was more prevalent than abundance, and body fat shielded from starvation.

By nature, women are especially designed to store energy in the form of fatty tissue, as they are designed to bear children and to breastfeed (formula feeding is a relatively recent invention). Fat is also more evenly spread on women's bodies. In men, it tends to concentrate around the abdomen (the famous 'beer belly' or 'pot belly'), which makes them more prone to heart attacks, as it is closer to the heart. Men are usually advised to lose weight for that reason.

Beauty ideals change throughout time and from one culture to another. In prehistoric times, obese women were considered beautiful and worshipped like goddesses, as shown by some ancient carvings of 'Earth Mothers'. In some African countries, obesity is a sign of abundance, something to be proud of, as it is a sign of success. In our society, the ideal of slimness was first created by fashion, movies and advertising. It then became a health issue. Nowadays, we don't just have to be skinny; we have to be fit as well. We need to have trim and muscular bodies, which puts us under even more pressure, which is detrimental, as it is a difficult goal to achieve. The pressure to be perfect causes unnecessary stress and makes us give up trying to lose weight altogether.

The middle-aged spread, beer gut, spare tyre or muffin top (there are lots of names for it and none are flattering) is a specific weight gain that seems to appear out of nowhere as we enter our thirties, forties and beyond. It's an accumulation of fat around the belly. Having a big middle seems to be an inevitable part of entering middle age. Even though it is preventable, it is one of the most common reasons for becoming overweight and failing to lose weight. It seems to be an insidious condition that creeps up on us while we're busy pursuing careers, rearing children and paying off mortgages.

Perhaps you too were slimmer in your younger years. Perhaps you've become less active physically, which means less muscle and less fat burning. Less hormones circulating in the bloodstream means energy tends to be conserved rather than used up. As you get older, you also tend to concentrate more on eating as a source of pleasure. Television programs encourage you to take up stylish cooking as a hobby. Celebrities show you how to create tasty meals that are superbly presented – mouth-watering stuff, impossible to resist!

But punishment follows your indulgence in such a seemingly harmless pursuit: kilograms slowly but surely pile up until you can't fit into your jeans any more. Only slim and juvenile looks obtain the seal of approval in society, so you feel old and fat, which is depressing. Your body feels stiff and sluggish, which doesn't make you want to move and exert yourself. You prefer to spend your leisure time in front of the TV with your favourite goodies. This is the 'couch potato' vicious cycle.

Bad habits are easy to make, but not easy to break. They take years to be established. Ask yourself *why* you want to complete this cycle now, *what* motivates you to end it and start anew. In my previous book, *The Magic of Willpower,* I explain this process in depth. Keep in mind all the reasons why you want to change. Don't deviate from your vision, your ultimate purpose. This mental imagery will drive you towards your goal.

Designed to cope with times of famines, your body is resistant to weight loss, as well as being genetically programmed to store fat as a sort of insurance policy against scarcity. Therefore, if you don't make a conscious decision to watch your food intake from an early age, probably as early as your late teens, you might end up overweight. There are some lucky people who have 'skinny genes' and never seem to put on weight, no matter what they eat. These are few and far between, but they also need to watch their food intake as their metabolism will slow down over time. Besides, they are not immune to diabetes and arteriosclerosis. However slim they look on the outside, a diet of junk food and soft drinks is sure to create havoc on the inside.

When you begin to control your diet, you may find that losing weight is more difficult than you expected. It might go well for a couple of weeks. The kilograms come off easily at the start. Then all of a sudden, *nothing*. The body has a tendency to maintain its present weight, the set point. When you reach a 'plateau' (when the scales stop moving), it means that your body has made adjustments in metabolism and fat storage, as well as in energy expenditure, to preserve its set point.

The body adapts to its new weight and sticks with it, and no matter what you do, it doesn't seem to make a difference. In fancy terms, this is called *adaptive thermogenesis* (thermo= heat and genesis= production). Calories can be burnt and converted to pure energy which is measured in terms of heat (it's the energy needed to raise the temperature of 1 gram of water by 1 degree Centigrade). When there is thermogenesis, your body adapts to a lower caloric intake by burning less energy. Creating a caloric deficit doesn't work any more.

Because of the set point, you may think that your body is working against you. You've done well for a while, but no matter how hard you try, the kilograms have stopped coming off. Don't despair if your weight has stabilised itself. This is your body's natural survival mechanism, and it's an effective way to cope with shortages that were so common throughout history and are still common in some parts of the globe. The set point is a weight that your body feels comfortable at and endeavours to maintain, even if it's not a healthy weight for you.

In the worst case scenario, your weight might even go up by two or three kilos. You can do a lot of different things to overcome a plateau: eating less, eating more, zigzagging your calories (eating a different amount of calories each day), fasting one day and eating normally the next, changing the type of exercise you do, having a 'free' day when you can eat what you want...

The secret is to give yourself more TIME. Be patient. Rushing weight loss might be more rewarding psychologically, because of the rapid results you obtain. But this quick euphoria can backfire, as your body reaches a point when it refuses to cooperate and stubbornly wants to remain at the same weight.

Your body is conditioned to maintain its current weight and even tends to put on *more* weight given the chance. If your set point is high and, if you keep eating without making any changes to your diet, it will remain high, and it might even get higher over time. Human bodies are programmed to put on weight rather than lose it. But if you are patient and persistent and continue to eat sensibly while being physically active, you will lose weight, and you will lower your set point. Not giving up is the answer, no matter how discouraged you are at times. Your endurance will be rewarded eventually.

Think of the set point as something you can work with, instead of working against it. Use it to your benefit. If you lower your set point, your body will tend to remain at that weight, which is great news. The longer you've been at a particular weight, the better your chances will be to maintain it effortlessly. Each time you reach a plateau, your weight will stagnate for a while before dropping any further. Losing weight is like going down steps, and while each step is a new set point, it is also a small victory for you. A new set point is a positive sign, an opportunity, not a setback. While it may seem annoying, it means that your diet is *working*.

The set point is a reliable mechanism, but it's also a double-edged sword. On the negative side, it will make you regain all the weight you've lost if you're not careful and veer away from your eating plan. On the positive side, it helps you keep your weight down. Once you've reached your optimum size and have maintained it for six to twelve months, your body's set point will begin working in your favour. It will enable you to remain at the same weight, once and for all without struggling.

If you happen to eat too much on the odd occasion, your body will burn off the excess calories instead of turning them into fat stores. You won't have to weigh yourself as frequently any more; maybe just once a month instead of every week. Your set point will regulate your weight automatically. You won't have to worry and you won't have to do anything drastic – simply maintain a sensible diet and lifestyle, with a reasonable level of physical activity. You will regain trust in your body and you will feel good about yourself.

Key Points and Strategies:

- Overcome your body's tendency to store fat
- Eat sensibly and be physically active
- Be patient and persistent when overcoming a plateau
- See a new set point is a positive sign, not a setback
- Trust the set point mechanism: it will help you maintain your new weight

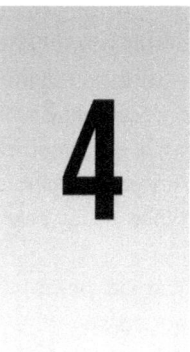

4

CARBOHYDRATES ARE GOOD FOR YOU

The difference between good and bad carbs is the difference between helpful and harmful. Good carbs will help you lose weight while feeling great.

Antonia, aged 53, has been told by her doctor that she needs to lose at least fifteen kilos for health reasons. She has been trying to lose weight for seven weeks, but nothing much has happened so far. Her diet just doesn't seem to work. Antonia is sure she's doing the right thing: she eats a lot of leafy salads with lemon juice and pepper, as well as lean meat and fish, steamed vegetables, natural low-fat yoghourt and NO bread, rice, pasta or potatoes. In the first two weeks of her diet, she lost two kilograms, but now it looks like her weight won't move any more.

Although she feels hungry, tired and irritable most of the time, Antonia is reluctant to give up her diet and resume her former eating pattern, which means no proper meals, but a lot of sugary and salty snacks throughout the day. Antonia feels guilty about eating sugar and gets bloated when she snacks all the time. She thinks that in order to lose weight, she needs to eliminate ALL carbohydrates from her diet. She thinks that a high protein diet is the only way to lose weight effectively, and she's actually read a number of bestselling books that confirm her belief.

Antonia is right about avoiding sugar and processed foods in general, as manufacturers add a lot of sugar and salt to them. Even fruit juice contains sugar in a concentrated form. But she's wrong to condemn carbohydrates altogether. Complex carbohydrates are good for you, especially if you want to lose weight. Carbohydrates are one of the three main macronutrients (fat and protein are the other two), and they are the body's preferred source of energy. They are not your enemies, but your allies!

What is body fat? It's one of the basic components of the structure of your body, along with water, muscle, bones, and organs such as your brain, liver, kidneys, stomach and pancreas. There are two types of fat: essential fat and storage fat. Both are necessary for healthy, normal body functions. Essential fat is distributed in different parts of your organism, such as bone marrow, internal organs, central nervous system and even muscles.

Women have a higher percentage of essential fat, which is necessary for the reproductive function. Storage fat is the one you accumulate under your skin and in certain areas of your body as well as in your muscles. It also protects your organs from injury, as it forms a sort of shield around them. Though it is desirable to have *some* storage fat, too much of it is unhealthy and leads to being overweight or obese.

A normal range of body fat for women is around 25%, and for men around 15% (more or less for both women and men, depending on age and level of fitness). Fat around the waist is worse than fat around your thighs and buttocks, as it increases your risk of diabetes, hypertension, heart disease, cancer and even dementia. *Storage fat* is what you need to reduce when deciding to lose weight.

Fat is not the static and sluggish mass we once thought it was. It plays an active and harmful role in the body, interfering with internal processes. Additional storage fat requires more oxygen and nutrients to live: blood vessels need to circulate more blood to the fat tissue, which increases the workload of the heart. Fatty deposits build up in arteries supplying the heart, clogging them up and increasing the likelihood of a heart attack.

Obesity is the major cause of type 2 diabetes. Normally it occurs in adults, but is now more and more frequently seen in children, which is alarming. Excessive storage fat can cause *resistance* to insulin, the hormone that regulates blood sugar. When obesity causes insulin resistance, blood sugar becomes elevated. This is dangerous, because high blood sugar causes long-term damage to the body. Blood sugar coats red blood cells, causing them to become stiff. These 'sticky cells' have lost their suppleness and agility, thus creating havoc with blood circulation, causing bad cholesterol to build up inside your blood vessels. This process can take months or even years before you feel anything. The fragile blood vessels in your eyes, kidneys and feet are the most susceptible, so problems are usually noticed in those areas first (like blurred vision or painful feet).

Insulin has been called the 'fat storage hormone'. Your body is a clever machine that can turn food into energy or fat, according to your needs and depending on the constant interaction of numerous substances in your body. What is the main role of insulin? It enables your body to absorb energy from carbohydrates (starch and sugar). *Glucose* delivers the energy you need to live, and it comes from the *carbohydrates* you eat. Blood sugar or blood glucose refers to sugar that is transported through the bloodstream to supply *energy* to all the cells in your body.

To use the glucose that your body obtains from carbohydrates, you need insulin, which is produced by the pancreas. Insulin allows the glucose in your blood to enter body cells and there it is burnt for processes requiring energy. Some of the glucose is stored in the liver for later use in the form of *glycogen*, an energy reserve that can be quickly mobilised to meet a sudden need for glucose. What can't be stored as glycogen, or immediately used, gets stored as fat. When there is an excessive amount of sugar in your bloodstream, some of it will automatically be converted to fat. In the case of insulin resistance, most of the glucose gets turned into fat because cells have become immune to the effect of this hormone. Soon you feel hungry again and crave sugar to compensate the glucose deficit in your bloodstream.

As your blood sugar rises after a meal, it triggers the release of insulin. Refined sugar enters the bloodstream almost immediately, followed by a quick and sharp rise in insulin. After the initial high, you begin to feel tired, dizzy, weak and light-headed, unable to perform demanding tasks, unable to concentrate properly and above all: you're HUNGRY. Refined sugar has hundreds of pseudonyms: dextrose, fructose, maltose, galactose, maltodextrin, corn syrup, high fructose corn syrup, malt syrup, rice bran syrup, brown molasses, fruit juice, golden syrup, treacle, concentrated fruit juice, honey – just to name a few.

Manufacturers change the name of sugar to give you the impression that a product is sugar-free, when it is actually high in sugar. Sugar is *addictive,* and it is added to many popular products, such as breakfast cereals, bread, soups and sauces. Our diet is full of refined, nutrient-depleted foods and contains on average twenty teaspoons of added refined sugar every day.

We eat as much sugar in two weeks as our grandparents did in a year.

Sugar is bad for you, not only for its effect on insulin production, but also because it accelerates the ageing process. It binds itself to proteins that are the building block of the skin and other tissues, in the form of elastin and collagen. Sugar also compromises the immune system, as it reduces the effectiveness of white blood cells.

Every time you eat sugar, your pancreas produces insulin to counteract its effect. If the pancreas is overworked, it leads to insulin resistance, a pre-cursor of diabetes: the pancreas slows down significantly, and diet and exercise need to be addressed very quickly to avoid full-blown diabetes. Some ethnic groups are more prone to diabetes type 2 than others, such as people of Asian, African and Mediterranean descent, as well as Aboriginal Australians and Native Americans.

A slim and fit person can tolerate the occasional sugary snack without any ill-effects, but overweight and obese people need to be extremely cautious with refined sugar. The more weight you carry, the more harmful sugar is for you. Sugar contributes to the vicious circle of starving for goodies, eating them, feeling better for a short time, only to feel sluggish and ravenous soon afterwards.

You swirl and swirl around, putting on more and more weight, as the excess glucose is stored in your fat cells. Sugar has a *rebound* effect and the cycle repeats itself, over and over. Sugar is *habit-forming.* You acquire a desire for the sweet taste that stimulates the pleasure centre in your brain. You eat it because your blood sugar is low most of the time, and you develop a craving for it. But the relief is short-lived.

Your body is in biological turmoil. No wonder your pancreas is likely to resign after working overtime, day after day! Artificial sweeteners are not the answer though, as they won't help you overcome your addiction to the sweetness of sugar foods. And it has even been proven that artificial sweeteners can still stimulate insulin production, thus promoting hunger like sugar does.

Today, most people agree that refined sugars are the 'bad guys', and they have been blamed for the obesity epidemic for good reason. Stay away from them if you want to lose weight or maintain your current shape.

The 'good guys' are the slow (=complex) carbohydrates found in wholegrain breads, pasta, brown rice, potato and sweet potato. Potatoes have been looked down upon since the seventies, but they have now regained their rightful place in a balanced diet, as they are packed with nutrients and fibre, as long as they're eaten with the skin on. Sweet potatoes are not necessarily better than white potatoes. As long as they're whole, unprocessed and part of a balanced meal, all potatoes are of value, in moderation. Avoid French fries and potato chips!

Slow carbohydrates have to be broken down into simple components before they can be absorbed, which is why they are also called complex carbohydrates. Your body takes a long time to process them, and uses energy in the process. As a result, energy is released *slowly* and *steadily* into your bloodstream, without the discomfort of a rapid spike followed by a steep drop. These are the carbohydrates that need to be part of a healthy diet, as they work like magic for weight loss.

When I recommend carbohydrates, it will *always* be complex carbohydrates, *never* refined sugar or manufactured products. Complex carbohydrates give you a constant supply of energy, and insulin production remains *constant*. This ensures an adequate blood sugar level, making you feel energetic and giving you a feeling of wellbeing. Complex carbohydrates raise your blood glucose level gradually, promoting the slow and steady release of insulin. They give you a unique feeling of lasting stamina and wellbeing, something you can't achieve with a diet based solely on salads, green vegetables, protein and fat.

When we are healthy, insulin acts as a blood sugar regulator, keeping our blood sugar at a comfortable level. Big fluctuations don't occur. A sensible diet derives 45 to 65 % of total daily calories from complex carbohydrates. Complex carbs include whole grains, brown rice, whole wheat pasta, legumes (beans and pulses), fruit and vegetables. Protein-rich foods should provide 10 to 35 % of your total daily calories, and fat approximately 20 to 35 %.

With a diet rich in complex carbohydrates, you tend to convert most of your calories into energy instead of storing them as fat. Most of the foods rich in complex carbohydrates are also rich in *fibre,* which is an advantage, as fibre slows the absorption of carbohydrates. A high fibre intake will make carbohydrates an even more efficient fuel. The higher in fibre, the better carbohydrate foods are for you.

The *Glycaemic Index* concept was introduced to help people recognise which carbohydrates were more beneficial to them, in order to prevent diabetes and other lifestyle diseases. Carbohydrate foods have different effects on blood glucose and insulin response depending on the rate of digestion. This rate of digestion depends on how much fibre the food contains, because it slows the absorption from your gut or intestine. But you also need to consider how much fibre your meal contains as a whole, and how much *protein* you eat at the same time as your starchy item.

The glycaemic index is a numeric value attached to each carbohydrate item. It's a good indication whether to make a certain item a regular part of your diet. But it doesn't give us all the answers to the equation of weight loss, and I won't turn it into the holy grail of dieting. Focus on the fibre content of each item, as well as the overall nutritious value of each meal, rather than becoming obsessed with a number which is only theoretical.

The glycaemic index measures how quickly your blood sugar rises after ingesting a particular carbohydrate. Each food is assigned a value from 0 -100, based on how fast blood sugar increases in the next two hours after consuming the starchy food. A value of 100 represents a food that raises your blood sugar very quickly, such as pure white sugar or a straight glucose drink. A value of 59 means your blood sugar response will be more moderate, as in the case of brown rice.

For blood glucose stabilisation, hunger prevention and weight loss, brown rice is a much better choice than pure white sugar or a glucose drink. Eating low GI foods during the day will suppress your appetite and provide stable, consistent energy levels, as blood sugar is better controlled. A sudden drop in blood sugar immediately makes you hungry.

Eating low GI foods means less of your calories will be stored as fat, and you will burn fat more easily. You won't overload your system with excessive amounts of simple carbohydrates or sugar that will immediately be converted to fat.

A low GI food is under 55, while a food under 70 is medium; anything above 70 is high and to be avoided. What you eat in conjunction with your carbs will affect the overall GI. When you eat a protein with your carbohydrate, the total GI value of your meal will decrease, since protein is a very complex molecule that will slow the digestion of your carbohydrate. Fats also have this effect, so including a small amount of fat with each meal is useful.

More important than the GI value is the amount of fibre in your foods, and whether they contain simple or complex carbohydrates. Avoid simple carbohydrates altogether if you want to slim down. In excess, even fruit can be harmful, although it is packed with fibre and nutrients. And it is certainly a better choice than concentrated fruit juice or manufactured sugary snacks.

It may be wise to consume fruit in moderation, up to three pieces a day. Even though they rank low on the GI scale, most types of fruit are high in glucose, a simple carbohydrate. Excessive glucose cannot be burnt up immediately and has to be stored in the liver as glycogen. If there is an excessive amount of glucose in your body, it will be stored as fat. To be on the safe side, limit yourself to two to three pieces or cups of fruit per day: e.g. an apple, a pear and an orange or: a cup of grapes and a cup of berries. Don't eat all your fruit allowance at once; preferably, stagger it throughout the day.

Most of the foods rich in complex carbohydrates are also rich in fibre, which is an advantage, as fibre slows the absorption of carbohydrates. A high fibre intake will make carbohydrates an even more efficient fuel for steady weight loss.

The higher in fibre it is, the better a carbohydrate food is for you. It keeps you full longer, preventing hunger. It gives you energy on a steady basis, without peaks and drops. It will help you lose weight as well as keep diabetes and high cholesterol at bay. Fibre will keep you regular, eliminating waste products and toxins from your body, as well as mopping up excess cholesterol from your bloodstream.

EXAMPLES OF HIGH FIBRE COMPLEX CARB FOODS

Breads	Serve	Carbohydrates (g)	Fibre (g)
Wholemeal	1 slice	13	1.8
Multigrain	1 slice	14	1.4
Rye bread, light	1 slice	14	1.8
Rye bread, dark	1 slice	14	2.8
Lebanese bread/Pita	50 g	25	1.2

Cereals	Serve	Carbohydrates (g)	Fibre (g)
Oat bran	2 tablespoons	8	2.4
Barley bran	2 tablespoons	9	2.3
Muesli	2 tablespoons	17	3
Rolled oats	¾ cup	19	2.5
Weet-bix	2 biscuits	19	3.6
Puffed wheat	1 ½ cup	22	2

Rice and Barley	Serve	Carbohydrates (g)	Fibre (g)
Rice, white, cooked	1 cup	42	1.2
Rice, brown, cooked	1 cup	48	2.4
Spaghetti, macaroni and fettuccine, white, cooked	1 cup	37	0.6
Wholemeal pasta, cooked	1 cup	37	1.5
Barley, pearled, raw	100 g	61	10

Brown rice is better than white rice: it has twice as much fibre and is a good source of vitamins and minerals. It contains B group vitamins as well as iron. White rice is okay when brown rice is not available (e.g. when you're eating out). Wholemeal (a.k.a. whole wheat) pasta is preferable to ordinary pasta as it is high in fibre, which slows the absorption of carbohydrates.

Vegetables	Serve	Carbohydrates (g)	Fibre (g)
Pumpkin	100 g	8	3.5
Parsnip	100 g	10	3
Potato, peeled	1 small	13	2.2
Potato, with skin	1 small	14	3.5
Sweet potato	100 g	17	2.4
Corn, cooked	½ cup	23	2

Banana

Unlike most other fruits that contain mainly fructose (simple carbohydrate), banana is full of starch (complex carbohydrate), while being high in fibre. Rich in pectin, banana is a super food that aids digestion and cleanses toxins from the body. It has vitamin B6, iron and potassium, while being low in salt. Banana increases calcium absorption, lowers blood pressure and protects against heart attack and stroke, as well as kidney and liver disease. Banana is high in nutrition, but not acid, and has a rather bland but pleasant taste. Mashed banana is an excellent starter food for babies when you introduce them to solids. Bananas have an average GI of 52, which is low (but it can be higher if your banana is over-ripe and very sweet).

Legumes

Legumes (a.k.a. pulses) include beans, soy beans, pinto beans, white beans, kidney beans, peas, chick peas, snap beans and lentils. They are full of fibre and most of their calories come from complex carbohydrates; they are digested slowly, keeping you satisfied longer. The complex carbs in legumes prevent insulin in the bloodstream from spiking and causing hunger. Legumes are extremely nutritious, high in protein but very low in fat. Their high fibre content helps reduce bad cholesterol. These high fibre foods may also prevent bowel cancer if eaten regularly. Legumes are rich in folic acid and Vitamin B6, as well as potassium and antioxidants. Research has shown that eating this 'super food' four or more times per week reduces the risk of heart disease while keeping you slim. Legumes are extremely versatile and cheap.

Soy beans contain valuable isoflavones that can mimic the effects of female hormones without negative side-effects. They can help alleviate the symptoms of premenstrual tension or menopause. Recent research has shown that more soy in the diet may prevent breast cancer. Soy products have caused controversy and people have been concerned about their effect on the body. But recent research has proven that soy provides a formidable defence against cardiovascular disease, certain forms of cancer in men and women, as well as osteoporosis. It I is also much more than just another type of oestrogen. Due to their selective mode of action utilising specific cell receptors, soy isoflavones promote beneficial oestrogen-like effects, without the harmful effects of conventional oestrogen replacement therapy.

Legumes	Serve	Carbohydrates (g)	Fibre (g)
Chick peas, cooked	100 g	22	6
Lentils, boiled	100 g	17	5
Three Bean Mix	100 g	14	4
White beans and Lima beans (cooked)	100 g	13	7.5
Baked beans in tomato sauce	100 g	11	7.3
Pease, fresh	100 g	8	4.5

Make complex carbohydrates your staple foods, so they can sustain you and give you energy throughout your busy day. Most diets have a high failure rate, because they restrict carbs too much. You end up worn out and constantly hungry. Hunger is a big hurdle for the dieter. It's probably the main reason why so many people can't stick to a weight loss program. The fear of being hungry can stop people from attempting to lose weight in the first place. They think they need to starve themselves in order to be thin. This is not true, as a diet rich in complex carbohydrates can normalise your blood sugar level and keep hunger to a minimum. Overweight and obese people produce too much insulin, which exacerbates hunger pangs. But once you lose weight and maintain a leaner body shape, your insulin production will revert to normal, and you won't feel so hungry all the time.

Your body is conditioned to put on weight. If you lose your kilos too quickly, you will regain them within a short period of time, and you will probably end up heavier than you were before. Your body gets the message that you're trying to starve it, and you feel exhausted and irritable, as well as ravenous. Your metabolism will slow down and fat burning almost ceases completely, as your body wants to preserve its fat stores.

Overproduction of insulin aggravates the problem, making it more difficult to lose weight. With your blood sugar level constantly fluctuating, your body has no choice but to go into starvation mode. You end up without energy and feeling more miserable by the day. There seems to be no way out.

Simply restricting your dietary intake is not enough. Even exercise doesn't always deliver the results you're hoping for. Over-exercising can also send your metabolism into starvation mode. Listen to your body carefully and acknowledge signs of fatigue. Recovery time is just as important as workout time. Keep your exercise sessions sweet and short, and don't push yourself too hard.

You can 'trick' your body into losing weight, with a diet rich in complex carbohydrates. These carbs must be as unrefined as possible and high in fibre. Your body won't go into starvation mode, and your metabolism won't slow down as it usually does on a restrictive diet. You can lose weight and feel terrific at the same time.

Should you go gluten-free?

Gluten is a *protein* found in wheat products such as breads and pasta, as well as in rye and barley. The only people who should stay clear of gluten are those with gluten intolerance: celiac disease or gluten sensitivity. Gluten in itself has no special health benefits. But all the wholegrain products that contain this protein are rich in complex carbohydrates, vitamins, minerals and fibre. As part of a balanced diet, wholemeal and whole grain foods may lower the risk of diabetes and heart disease and even some forms of cancer. Replacements for these foods have become easier to find in supermarkets, but remain expensive for people on a limited budget.

Less than one percent of the population has *celiac disease*, a condition caused by an abnormal immune response to gluten. It can damage the lining of the small intestine, which can prevent important nutrients from being absorbed. Some common symptoms are bloating, gas, constipation, diarrhoea, anaemia, bone pain, joint pain, headaches, fatigue, depression, irritability, itchy skin rash and infertility. A lot of people with the disease don't have any symptoms at all, although they tend to feel generally unwell. To find out if you have celiac disease, you need a blood test.

If you have *non-celiac gluten sensitivity,* your body reacts adversely if you ingest products that contain gluten. It's not an immune response, but rather a *stress* reaction. Symptoms are not well-defined.

A hoard of physical complaints has been linked to gluten intolerance:

- Digestive issues such as gas, bloating, acid reflux, constipation or diarrhoea
- Fatigue, dizziness, lethargy, fainting spells and even death
- Hormone imbalances such as premenstrual tension or unexplained infertility
- Migraine or tension headaches, neck and back pain
- Mood swings, anxiety, insomnia, hyperactivity, inability to concentrate, depression and suicide
- Chronic fatigue or fibromyalgia (unexplained tiredness and pain)
- Inflammation and swelling of joints in fingers, elbows, knees or hips

This is a scary list. With a hectic schedule and daily exposure to chemicals in the environment, more and more people develop sensitivities and allergies. Stress can make you react adversely to something you could previously to tolerate without discomfort. This is one of the reasons gluten-free diets have become so popular. People want to find a solution to feeling unwell, and it's worth trying anything that could possibly make a difference.

There is no blood test to determine if you are gluten sensitive. The only way to find out is to do an *elimination* diet: you take it out of your diet for two to three weeks before reintroducing it. If you notice that your symptoms subside and you feel much better without gluten, and feel worse again after you've reintroduced it, you may well be gluten intolerant. The only thing to do is to eliminate if from your diet completely. Even a small amount can cause a negative reaction in your body. From now on, read labels carefully, as a lot of processed foods, and even medications and supplements may contain gluten.

Key Points and Strategies:

- Avoid simple carbohydrates like sugar, honey or corn syrup
- Eat food rich in complex carbohydrates: breads and cereals, rice, pasta, carbohydrate rich vegetables (e.g. pumpkin and sweet potato), bananas and legumes (e.g. peas, beans and lentils)
- Eat wholemeal products whenever possible: wholemeal bread and rolls, brown rice, wholemeal pasta
- Eat fibre to increase the beneficial effect of carbohydrates
- Use the Glycaemic Index (GI) as a good indicator whether a carb is good for you, but don't treat it as the holy grail of weight loss. What's more important is the overall nutritional value of your meal, including its fibre and protein content
- Remember that a gluten-free diet is not necessary, unless you have celiac disease or gluten sensitivity.

5

SEROTONIN, THE NATURAL 'FEEL-GOOD' SUBSTANCE

Serotonin improves your wellbeing!

For Caroline, aged 36, eating and stress are interrelated. Her fridge and pantry are filled with goodies; food is always accessible. It's her safety valve when she feels frustrated and about to explode. She believes it's her only source of pleasure. To her, life without salt and vinegar chips, jelly beans and Mars bars is not worth living.

With three young children and a husband who works away, she feels a big weight on her shoulders. Even though she loves her children, she often feels overwhelmed and under pressure, resentful for not being able to relax and do the things she enjoys, such as reading and listening to music.

Looking after small children is one of the most demanding jobs in the world. Twenty-four hours a day, seven days a week, a mother has to be there, and is expected to be always patient, loving and supportive. Society expects stay-at-home mums like Caroline to be perfect in every sense, with a spotless house, manicured garden, and well-behaved and well-groomed children.

But she doesn't get paid for all her hard work, and receives little recognition and support. She often feels isolated and, even though she loves her family, she secretly longs for the single life she was leading before settling down. For reasons that may differ due to their circumstances, many people feel a pervasive sense of loneliness and a silent despair that eats away at them. Their only escape is to find solace in food.

There may be hope for you if you suffer from stress – and who doesn't? The right food can help you relax without making you fat. From the day you were born, you were programmed to enjoy eating; it was necessary for your survival. But over the years, food has become a substitute for something missing in your life. You still want to enjoy eating, but not at the cost of being overweight or obese. You also want to enjoy being slim: this has become a priority for you.

Food is a source of energy. If you don't need it, your body will store it as fat, and you will gain weight as a result. Sounds simple... so why do we eat so much? Why can't we resist the sight or smell of delicious food or the crunchiness of our favourite snack? Why do we feel unhappy, frustrated, irritable, depressed or angry when we attempt to reduce our food intake? Is food some kind of drug? In a sense it is, because it influences the way chemicals interact in your body. In your brain, *neurotransmitters* act like messengers that carry instructions to different cells. There are over 100 different neurotransmitters in the brain alone, and *serotonin* is one of them. Overweight people have too much insulin, but they also lack serotonin, which exacerbates hunger and cravings.

Serotonin acts like an antidepressant, a natural mood enhancer, and its production is activated when you're eating. This is one of the reasons why eating is so pleasurable, apart from the taste bud experience. One of the objectives of sensible dieting is to keep your insulin levels constant, without notable spikes. The other objective is to promote a steady level of serotonin in your brain to prevent hunger attacks and cravings. Serotonin reduces your desire for food in the absence of hunger – that is, when you suddenly feel an urge to eat something, even though you're not really hungry.

A carbohydrate-rich diet will make you feel full and it will boost your serotonin levels. You won't be tempted to overeat, as you will feel satisfied most of the time. Hunger weakens your determination, and it can literally drive you insane! Hunger can easily trigger a binge. Research has shown that people who binge have extremely low serotonin levels. A carbohydrate-rich diet can be useful to alleviate stress and to prevent cravings.

Sadly, negative attitudes towards overweight people have taken root in modern society, and many people think that fat people are lazy. In reality, most overweight people are workaholics and perfectionists who rarely grab the opportunity to get in touch with their true selves. They tend to sacrifice themselves for other people. They often don't take time to look after themselves properly and to have fun. And when everything gets too much and they feel out of control, they turn to food, their best friend and comforter.

Food takes away stress and can help you overcome unwelcome feelings, such as loneliness, boredom and fatigue. Nothing beats a chocolate bar when you're feeling low... You can eat without harming anyone except *yourself*, as guilt kicks in eventually, and you feel unhappy and worthless because you're 'too fat'. To forget about it and feel better, you fetch another tub of ice cream from the freezer!

If you understand how serotonin makes you feel better, and how carbohydrates can help your brain produce it, you can use this knowledge to your advantage. You won't need to self-medicate your emotional stress with food any more. Serotonin is a natural 'drug', produced by your own body and always available from the right fuel: carbohydrates. The less *protein* you eat with your carbohydrate meal, the higher your serotonin production will be.

Cut down on protein-rich foods any time you need the *full* serotonin effect; it will be the equivalent of taking an antidepressant or a sedative. Protein-rich foods include lean meat, fowl, fish, seafood, eggs and low-fat dairy products. Legumes like peas, beans, lentils and chick peas are rich in both complex carbohydrates and vegetable protein. Their advantage is that the protein they contain won't hamper serotonin production. Eat them in combination with vegetables and complex carbs like brown rice and whole meal bread or pasta.

Do you believe you can't go without sugar? Do you eat while under stress or when feeling overwhelmed? Sugar helps you produce serotonin, the 'happy substance', which relaxes you. Subconsciously you know this, and this is why you reach for the cookie jar when things are getting on top of you. When your brain lacks serotonin, you feel nervous, anxious, uneasy and insecure. Your instinct tells you that something sweet will make you feel better. It usually works, but for a limited time only, until the cycle starts all over. Feeling yuck, craving sugar, feeling better and feeling yuck again...

So far, no one has been able to fully understand the body's complex chemistry. Many different hormones and numerous other substances influence how we feel; some of them are neurotransmitters. A neurotransmitter is a chemical involved in the transmission of nerve impulses between nerve cells; serotonin is one of them. This substance is formed in your brain but can also be found in other parts of your body, in particular, the lining of your digestive system. In the brain, serotonin plays a major role in regulating mood. It also gives you that feeling of satisfaction you experience after ingesting food. Serotonin is not only important to control your appetite, but it also promotes wellbeing, relaxation and is essential for a good night's sleep.

Carbohydrate meals help increase serotonin levels. Simple carbohydrates are temporarily effective at lifting your mood. This is why you crave sugar when you're feeling stressed or depressed. But sugar is not recommended as a regular part of any diet, due to its detrimental effect on insulin production, and rebound hunger effect. Luckily complex carbohydrates are effective at stimulating serotonin production, but only if eaten with small or moderate amounts of protein.

To maintain the desired serotonin effect, have a healthy carbohydrate snack every four hours: a banana, a cup of air-popped popcorn, a cup of cooked instant oatmeal porridge with fruit, two egg whites (or a little low-fat cottage cheese) on whole meal toast or gluten free crackers, raw carrots with spicy tomato dip, steamed corn on the cob. To have regular snacks is especially important if you're studying or involved in a task that demands a high level of concentration.

To feel relaxed and focused, I sometimes have a plate of wholemeal pasta and vegetables for lunch, without meat but with a sprinkle of low-fat grated cheese. The serotonin effect usually lasts me for the rest of the day. I don't get hungry until dinner time, and I am more patient with my family.

Because we live in a stressful world, it's useful to be aware that food can influence the way you feel and the way you cope with what life throws at you. Serotonin is a neurotransmitter that will make you feel cool, calm and collected as well as optimistic. With little or almost no protein added to your complex carbohydrate meal, you will feel the full impact of it, and you will find that it can work like magic to help you cope with your daily challenges. Eating is a biological process and it involves serotonin. A lack of this essential neurotransmitter will not only leave you hungry; you will be irritable, depressed and unable to deal with difficult issues.

In 'The Magic of Willpower' I explain that, in the mind, thoughts are translated into feelings. By changing your thoughts, you can change the way you feel. One way to influence your thought processes is through your diet: as you feel better physically, you will feel better mentally. The brain receives feedback from your body, and turns these messages into thoughts of wellbeing or discomfort. Serotonin could be one of the secrets to a healthy mind, and only carbohydrate foods can increase the production of this powerful substance.

Prozac, a popular anti-depressant of the SSRI family (Selective Serotonin Reuptake Inhibitors), works by increasing serotonin concentration in the brain. One of its side-effects is weight loss, due to decreased hunger and appetite. Maybe it's because you don't need to eat so much when you feel better. But, to experience wellbeing you don't need to take drugs. Consider these as a last resort, or if you suffer from severe depression. Avoid chemicals unless you've been diagnosed with an illness. It's safer to use complex carbohydrates to improve your mood and energy levels.

Key Points and Strategies:

- Alleviate stress by eating 'good' carbs: stick to complex carbohydrates, while avoiding simple carbohydrates like sugar and refined products
- Use serotonin to prevent hunger attacks and curb your appetite

- Use serotonin as a natural antidepressant, a 'feel good' substance
- Eat a carbohydrate-rich diet to boost your serotonin levels
- Add protein in moderation to your meal in order to maximise the relaxing 'serotonin effect'

6

HUNGER AND WILLPOWER

Don't starve yourself!

Courtney, 34, is in a relationship and has two children. She is overweight, with a BMI of 27, and has been trying to lose weight for the last five years with varying results. When she finally manages to drop a dress size, she is ecstatic, but her elation is short-lived. After being on a diet for a couple of months, she just gets *too* hungry. Tired of having to struggle all the time, she ends up giving in to her cravings for sugary and fatty foods, such as fried chicken, French fries, chocolate and cheesecake.

Courtney knows the caloric content of almost every food, and her bookshelf displays an impressive collection of diet books. She buys magazines just for their diet section and loves 'before and after' stories of big people who have lost a lot of weight. She subscribes to online diet and fitness newsletters, blogs and forums. She watches YouTube videos on how to lose weight. She has an app on her IPhone to count calories, another one to monitor her weight loss progress, as well as several fitness apps.

She has tried almost every new diet and religiously attends a weight loss club every week.

In spite of her determination, her persistence and her sincere desire to lose weight, Courtney's efforts seem to be in vain. 'I can't lose weight,' she says. And she believes it's because she doesn't have enough willpower. But her track record show that she has a lot of staying power, as she sticks with her resolutions for a long time, before the overwhelming urge to overeat takes hold of her again.

Courtney feels depressed and discouraged, as she hasn't been able to vanquish the long-time enemy that's been undermining her weight loss attempts: HUNGER.

Self-control is the mountain you need to climb, and if anything is in its way, get rid of it. If hunger is in its way, eliminate it. Hunger may be genuine, or it may just be a desire to eat: your mouth or brain telling you to ingest something in order to satisfy an urge. It may be just a habit, an addictive response. 'I'm hungry' often means: 'I want to put some food in my mouth.' Is it your head or your body that needs refueling?

True hunger can make you moody, irritable, irrational, angry and unable to concentrate. A little hunger can be healthy, especially before a meal, but intense hunger will make you put the first thing you see into your mouth. Intense hunger doesn't feel good. Health professionals hand out diet plans, books suggest food restrictions and companies even deliver calorie-controlled meals to your door to coerce you into losing weight. But no one seems to worry how you will feel and what you will do when you get hungry.

It's easy to say 'Eat this', 'Eat that' or 'Just stick with this plan.' How can you keep it up, with such tiny portions for each meal, especially when you've always been a big eater with a huge appetite? You feel miserable at the mere thought of being deprived and suffering. Hunger is painful, and who wants to suffer in order to attain a goal? A small amount of discomfort is acceptable, but to be miserable day after day is too much to handle for most people so they give up.

Hunger is a feeling of discomfort and weakness caused by a lack of food, coupled with a strong urge to eat. Hunger robs you of your energy: you can't focus, you're anxious and lethargic, and you can't work effectively. You slow down your movements and efforts, in an attempt to preserve energy. Hunger is a depressant, and it also causes insomnia. Try going to sleep on an empty stomach: it's almost impossible, even if you feel exhausted. Who wants to face sleepless nights for the sake of losing weight? The next morning you're worn out, but you force yourself to continue with your diet. You feel even more miserable. The cycle repeats itself unless you break it by breaking your diet. Hunger is not just a mental thing like a simple desire or a craving for a particular food. Hunger is a physical phenomenon, and it's not something you can easily ignore or talk yourself out of.

No one can endure starvation for more than a week or two, so you give up and blame yourself for not being superhuman. Most diets instruct you to count calorie or 'points', based on a food exchange lists. This seems reasonable at first glance, but these programs tend to be too restrictive and fail to provide you with enough fuel. You end up hungry and tired. These diets also deplete your brain of serotonin, turning you into a nervous wreck in no time. A binge on forbidden foods, high in 'empty calories', is just around the corner.

Stop using willpower to overcome hunger. Instead of starving yourself, give your body enough fuel in the form of complex carbohydrates, lean protein and reasonable amounts of fat.

Always eat when you feel hungry. Your body is not your enemy, but your ally. It's the only one you've got, so look after it! Be good to your body and satisfy its need for fuel and nourishment. Allow yourself to get slightly hungry before meals, so that you can learn to identify your personal hunger signals. But once you know you're hungry, there is only one thing to do: eat!

The key to sound eating habits and natural, permanent weight loss lies in your ability to recognise hunger and do something about it. The opposite of hunger is fullness or satiety. When you eat, aim at feeling full, but not *too* full. Aim at feeling 80 % satisfied: leave a little room for more at the end of each meal.

Some people who have been slim all their lives won't understand what the fuss is about. They do it naturally: they feel hungry, eat and stop as soon as they feel full. For overweight people it may not be so simple. In most cases, they are overweight because they eat too much. They have lost a natural instinct: the ability to interpret the body's signals of hunger and satiety. They may not even know that they've got such a clever in-built mechanism.

Hunger and fullness go hand in hand; like feeling tired, sleeping and waking up refreshed. You can't experience fullness unless you've experienced hunger, so avoiding it completely is not the solution. Hunger can be quite pleasant when you know you'll soon have something to eat. You won't put on weight by satisfying your natural instinct and being in tune with your body.

Don't be afraid to get hungry. Intense hunger is awful, and doesn't feel good. But mild to moderate hunger is normal and even healthy, and it's something you can allow yourself to experience three to four times a day. It's a signal that your metabolism is working, that you're burning the calories from your previous meal as well as dipping into your fat stores. It's a signal that it's time to refuel your body for the next few hours. If you always eat routinely, on a fixed schedule, you probably don't experience *real* hunger, and it could be a sign that you eat excessively.

Don't starve, but pay attention to the physical sensations of hunger. Real hunger is stomach hunger and it involves a complex interaction between your digestive system, your endocrine glands and your brain. You feel fatigued and find it hard to focus on a task. Your stomach aches and rumbles. Stomach noises can be quite loud! When you start eating in response to these sensations, you really enjoy your food: anything tastes glorious, and you immediately begin to feel better, both physically and mentally. Your bodily needs are being met and, every time this happens, a feeling of wellbeing ensues.

If you ignore stomach hunger, the symptoms will intensify. Your stomach begins to hurt quite badly. You find it even more difficult to concentrate and feel lightheaded or even dizzy. You might become irritable and cranky. No wonder 'hunger' and 'anger' sound similar! You may get a headache, and you may experience shakiness and nervousness. Now that you're ravenous, you're in danger of over-eating. The fullness signal in your brain will be bypassed as soon as you put something in your mouth. Now you're most likely to be out of control and binge.

In the ideal case scenario, you eat four times a day but each time, you wait until you feel *real* stomach hunger. You eat until satisfied then wait to be hungry again. This is the hunger-fullness cycle, when you're tuned into your body and its needs. Hunger and fullness are regulated by the *hypothalamus,* a small portion of the brain with several important functions in the nervous and endocrine system. One of its roles is to control food and water intake, hunger and thirst.

When you've had enough to eat, signals reach the hypothalamus to register fullness. When you're in tune with your body, you're able to recognise when it's time to stop eating. Your stomach feels *comfortable* but not over-stretched. You feel relaxed, more alert and have more energy. It takes twenty minutes for satiety signals to be processed by the brain. When you eat too fast without paying attention, you bypass this system and eat more than your body's caloric requirements.

Chronic dieting and yoyo dieting confuse your body's ability to regulate hunger and fullness. You end up not knowing whether you're hungry or not, due to the unnatural way you've been eating. You can't recognise the symptoms any more, because you've been overriding these signals for so long. But it doesn't take long to recover and soon you will be able to interpret your body's messages again and respond to them adequately.

Overweight people often have an insulin disturbance, which exacerbates hunger and compels them to eat more frequently and to consume bigger portions than people within the healthy BMI range. The bigger your body, the bigger its energy requirements; as you slim down, you will notice that you won't need to eat as much any more.

You may not always eat out of hunger. There are hundreds of reasons to put food in your mouth: boredom, stress, anxiety, fatigue, insecurity, feeling empty and unfulfilled, or simply out of habit. You eat without hunger and put on weight. Then you go on a diet and hunger without eating. You get told to stick to a strict eating plan, so you remain hungry after ingesting ridiculously small portions, thinking it's the right thing to do. But you do yourself damage, by ignoring your hunger and fullness signals.

Learn to recognise your own hunger signals. Hunger is subjective, and everyone feels it differently. Your goal is to be *free* of hunger most of the day, except for a reasonable period of time before a meal or a snack (20-30 minutes at the most). Maybe you're afraid of hunger; maybe you're afraid that you won't be able to stop eating once you give in to it. Develop a more constructive relationship with your hunger. Hunger tells you *when* you need food and *how much* of it. Instead of fearing it, make it your inner guide to healthy, safe, and satisfying eating.

To overcome your fear of hunger and identify its signals, use a hunger assessment scale from one to five – one being the absence of hunger, and two to five describing its intensity, when it is present and you can feel it.

HUNGER ASSESSMENT SCALE

1. **Not hungry**: feeling of fullness, contentment, wellbeing.
2. **A little hungry**: slight discomfort, mild desire for food, desire for more food after a meal.
3. **Hungry**: clear signs of hunger: weakness, rumbling stomach, strong desire for food.
4. **Very hungry:** strong signs of hunger: total lack of energy, inability to concentrate, dizziness, irritability.
5. **Extremely hungry:** signs of starvation: physical and mental suffering, obsession with food which permeates the mind and takes over everything else.

Level one, the absence of hunger, is not a problem, unless you're tempted to eat for reasons other than hunger: to cope with stress or reward the pleasure centres in your brain with sugary treats. My book 'The Magic of Willpower' contains strategies to overcome urges and resist temptation. It helps you deal with slip-ups, and how to overcome obstacles and remain motivated. The secret is to keep your goal in mind at all times, a constant reminder of where you're heading. A slip-up is not a failure, as it takes practice and persistence to develop healthy eating habits.

Don't allow yourself to reach hunger level four or five. If you do, it means you haven't been eating enough (or enough nutritious food) and your body requires more energy to function. If you're extremely hungry or starving, your brain won't be able to fulfil its task of analysing, memorising and coming up with solutions. It won't be able to fire impulses to activate every moving part of your body. The brain is a creative organ, a sophisticated computer. There is almost no limit to what it can do – but not without food! Brain cells require twice as much energy as other body cells.

Neurons are cells that communicate with each other. Always in a state of metabolic activity, they have a high demand for energy. Neurons manufacture *enzymes* and *neurotransmitters*, as well as being responsible for the bioelectric signals to enable communication throughout the nervous system. This nerve transmission alone consumes one-half of the brain's energy. The brain needs glucose. But too much glucose at once in the form of sugar or refined carbohydrates can actually deprive the brain of its main energy source. Complex carbohydrates are the solution, as they are time-release capsules of sugar for your brain: long-lasting energy, so you can work on a project for a long time without losing your focus.

Whenever you feel hungry, before, after and in between meals, make a note of it. Your ultimate goal is to be free of hunger, except for a short while before meals. To experience level two hunger from time to time is normal, even after you've eaten. It means you have room for some more food like a dessert. Consider it to be healthy, as you're adjusting to a new eating pattern. You don't need to do anything about level 2. Remind yourself that it will soon be time to eat again. Looking forward to your next meal will give you the reassurance that this feeling is transitory. When you begin eating, it can take a while before satiety kicks in, especially if you're used to stretching your stomach with big portions. Adjusting to normal portions doesn't take long, only a few days at the most as your stomach shrinks accordingly.

Once you reach level three, take action as soon as possible. Plan something healthy and nutritious in advance, so when you reach this level, you won't be caught unawares. Planning is the secret to successful weight loss. You risk over-eating or resorting to take-away meals, if you haven't planned in advance. This planning shouldn't take up too much time and energy. Keep it simple and give yourself several alternatives that you can store in containers in the fridge or freezer, and take with you when you're away from home.

While level three may be desirable up to 30 minutes before a meal, avoid levels four and five at all cost. When you're ravenous, you risk losing control over your food intake. It has been proven that food restriction sets the scene for the next binge, as it produces intense hunger. You eat nothing or very little all day long, come home in the evening and have a big binge. There are different reasons why people overeat. It can be for comfort and to relieve emotional pain or anxiety, but it can also be simply because they've allowed themselves to become too hungry.

Eat enough to feel satisfied, while keeping room for some more. Eat enough to avoid reaching levels 4 or 5. You can experience level 3, as long as the next meal is no further than half an hour away.

Extract from Courtney's food diary:

Friday, March 5th	Food consumed	Hunger level
07.00		2
07.30	Slice of wholemeal toast with two egg whites, grilled tomato and black coffee.	1
10.15		3
10.30	One apple.	3

12.00		4
12.30	Lentil burger, two carrot and two celery sticks.	2
14.00		3
15.00	Plain yoghourt (sugar free), blueberries and a few almond flakes.	2
18.00		4
18.45	Tomato, cucumber, capsicum and spring onion salad, steamed fish and broccoli.	2

Courtney's eating plan looks healthy and sensible: she has four meals with vegetables, fruit and quality protein. Every day was based on this principle, but, as she's reducing her food intake drastically, Courtney is not giving her body enough energy. She is sabotaging her diet by allowing herself to get too hungry. The following week, she decides to change her approach and included more carbs in her eating plan.

Wed, March 12th	Food consumed	Hunger level
07.00		2
07.30	Baked beans on two slices of wholemeal bread, porridge with sugar free applesauce.	1
10.15		2
10.30	One apple and one banana.	1
12.15		3
12.30	Salad with tomato, cucumber, carrot, capsicum, spring onion, green beans, corn and tuna. One tablespoon of olive oil and balsamic vinegar. Brown rice.	1

15.00		2
15.30	Two Weet-Bix, plain yoghourt (sugar free), strawberries and pine nuts.	1
18.30		2
19.00	Lean beef, steamed cauliflower, sweet potato, skinny white sauce with herbs.	1

This weight loss plan works better for Courtney, as she's not starving herself any more. She only gets hungry before meals, and only up to level three. She finds her meals pleasant and satisfying. Even though her weight loss may be slow to begin with and she may reach a few plateaus before attaining her goal, she will end up losing her excess weight, and maintain her new shape without struggling.

When you're hungry, do something about it. Give your body food, as long as it's the right kind of food: whole food – not processed, pre-packaged sugary, salty and fatty snacks, empty calories devoid of essential nutrients. Choose products that are high in complex carbohydrates. Choose product that are high in fibre. Choose products that are low in sugar and moderately low in fat. The sugar/fat combination is irresistible (hence our passion for chocolate) but ultimately, we're responsible for our choices.

We can't fix the world's problems, but we can do something about the food we eat! Stick to whole foods three to six times a day: fresh fruit and vegetables, complex carbohydrates, lean protein, and moderate amounts of healthy fat. At the same time, quit snacking on processed foods, and you will lose weight. The snacking habit has become engrained in society, with the abundance of take-away foods and supermarket convenience foods. After eating a balanced diet for some time, you'll stop craving these empty calories.

Wholesome food satisfies your body's need for nourishment, but it may take some time before the feeling of satiety sets in. Be patient, and suddenly you will think, 'This is a miracle. I've eaten a normal portion, and for the first time, I'm not hungry.' What's a normal portion? Clasp your hands together to form a small ball: this is the size of a healthy stomach. But this organ is highly adaptable and able to contain bucket loads of food! You can stretch your stomach by overloading it, but you will suffer the consequences: next time you eat you will want to stretch it again. As you reduce your portions, your stomach will shrink, and you will feel satisfied with less food.

How can you tell you're full? When you take a headache tablet, you don't expect it to work right away. You give it at least 20 to 30 minutes to be effective. Do the same when you're eating, as your brain needs some time to process the information that your 'fuel tank' has been replenished. With complex carbohydrates, it may take even longer than usual to feel satisfied, as you're not used to them, while possibly craving a sugar fix.

Give yourself the chance to experience the mental and physical satisfaction that comes from eating a diet moderately low in fat, high in fibre and high in complex carbohydrates. Instead of feeling heavy, bloated and lethargic, you will feel alert and energetic (full of beans!)

In case you're still genuinely hungry after a meal, have some more vegetables or salad. No one has ever become overweight or obese from eating excessive amounts of fresh tomatoes, capsicum, carrots, Brussels sprouts, broccoli or spinach leaves!

Appetite is more a desire than a genuine need for food. It often starts in the mind: you see a picture of a tantalising dish in a magazine or online. You see a brightly-coloured packet of cookies. You smell hot bread, roast chicken or Asian stir-fry while strolling down the shopping mall. You become hungry, or convince yourself that you are, as you want to reward the pleasure center in your brain. You begin eating and keep putting food into your mouth. It tastes so nice! You can't stop even though you know you're full. Something takes hold of you and you lose control.

You loathe wasting food, while other people in the world are starving. Some countries were poor not so long ago, but they now have an obesity problem too! As these nations become more developed, people give up wholesome traditions, subscribing to a Western lifestyle, with an explosion of processed foods available in brand new supermarkets and foreign-owned fast food chains. Mexico is a prime example: 50 % of its population is now obese, and the nation's government is concerned about the burden this represents to the health system. Emerging economies like India, China and Brazil are experiencing similar trends. By the way, Mexico is the biggest consumer of soft drink per capita in the world!

To avoid eating when you're full, it may be wiser to eat only one-course meals. A three-course meal with entrée and dessert will stimulate your taste buds, due to alternating flavours (sour, spicy, sweet…) that increase your appetite. You're likely to eat more and put on more weight. One-course meals are a lot safer to control an appetite that is 'out of control'.

Five small meals are usually better than three big ones. They are more likely to satisfy you and provide you with a constant supply of fuel throughout the day. Dividing your food allowance into several meals is psychologically more rewarding. It gives you the impression that you're eating more, as you're eating more often. Regular small meals will prevent cravings, while stimulating your metabolism: you will burn more calories and fat. Some people feel more comfortable with three meals, out of habit or convenience, or because it makes them feel more in control. If you need massive amounts of willpower to stop eating every time you sit down for a meal, you may benefit from having only three meals a day instead of five.

You can choose how many meals you want to have, according to your needs, habits and lifestyle. Allow yourself to be flexible with mealtimes. If you decide to skip a meal because you're not hungry, plan ahead: if you intend to go out, take a healthy snack with you, like a banana, an apple or some strawberries with a tub of plain yoghourt. If hunger catches up, this is better than buying a fast food. Alternatively, prepare your lunch or dinner in advance, and take it with you in a sealed container. You may not be hungry right now, but you will be later. Temptation may get hold of you if you don't prepare yourself. Planning is the secret to success.

If you think you can't resist a delicious food because you're afraid to miss out, tell yourself that many opportunities to eat a similar dish will arise in the future. You can say no today, but you can say yes tomorrow, if you wish to. And if you are hungrier tomorrow, it will taste even better.

Maybe you've tried everything to lose weight without success, so you believe you lack willpower. If you believe that you were born that way, let me assure you that willpower is not a genetic trait. It is not something that is given to certain people at birth while others miss out. Everyone *has* willpower. If you didn't have any, you wouldn't be able to perform the simplest tasks, like choosing your clothes or brushing your teeth. Unless you suffer from severe depression, you are capable of using willpower in your daily life.

Willpower is the ability to choose one course of action over another. It means either doing something ('green light') or deciding not to do it ('red light'). Willpower tells you to go or to stop, and you translate these commands into actions. Some actions are automatic, some are instinctive, some arise from your emotions (e.g. joy or sadness), and some are the result of an informed decision. Your intellect or common sense enables you to analyse a situation and decide which will be the best course of action. Willpower is the power to exert your will as a free individual, responsible and aware of the consequences of your actions.

Everything you do is proof that you have at least some degree of willpower. Without it, you wouldn't be able to live as a productive human being. You wouldn't be able to work or look after your children. You wouldn't be able to tend to your garden or pets. You wouldn't be able to perform simple chores around the house. As you go about your day, opportunities for choices arise, starting from the moment you wake up. Will you press the snooze button or get out of bed right away? Every day, your ability to choose proves that you *do* have willpower, even though you may believe otherwise.

You can use willpower to force yourself to do something you don't want to do. But it is a lot easier to use willpower to do something you *want* to do. If you really want to lose weight and are prepared to eat healthy, you will feel so good that you will want to continue eating that way. You hate being hungry and you hate feeling deprived, even for a limited time. You get so frustrated that all you want to do is eat, eat, and eat, regardless of the consequences. You want to make up for all the scrumptious food you've missed out on.

Willpower is self-discipline. If you didn't have any, you wouldn't be able to complete the simplest task, like unloading the dishwasher or brushing your teeth. You have enough self-discipline to read this book. Maybe you don't know yet how to discipline yourself with food. Self-discipline is like a muscle: the more you exercise it, the stronger it becomes. Every time you say 'no' to a food item that is full of calories but devoid of nutrients, and you eat a healthy alternative instead, you've demonstrated your ability to discipline yourself. You've done it once, so you can do it again. Every single step on your journey is a small victory.

Every time you're tempted to eat when you're not genuinely hungry, treat yourself to something else. Have a bubble bath, do some meditation, listen to music, read a page turner, or watch your favourite movie or TV show. Use your imagination and creativity to do anything that gives you joy and takes your mind off eating. Start a new hobby, write a blog, learn a new skill… Keeping yourself occupied with something pleasurable *but not edible* will divert your attention from food. Visualise your destination, and imagine already being there. Feel the feeling of having succeeded, and you will be halfway there.

If you starve yourself, your metabolism will slow down. Rather than burning energy, your body will conserve it. If you lose weight while on a drastic diet, you will soon regain it. Once you revert to your former eating habits, all the energy you consume will be turned into fat. If you starve yourself, you will program your body to put on *more* weight. With more fat stored, your body is now ready for the next crash diet. Your body is your best friend, but you wouldn't do this to your worst enemy!

A slow but steady weight loss guarantees long-term success. While quick results may be encouraging, they generally don't last very long. Fat can take a long time to burn, and if you lose weight too quickly, you can assume that you've mainly lost water. On top of that, rapid weight loss causes your metabolism to slow down, as you need to reduce your caloric intake dramatically. A slow weight loss will stop your from losing muscle, and it will prevent your skin from loosening, giving it plenty of time to contract and adjust to your new shape. A slow weight loss keeps fatigue and weight loss-related health problems at bay (e.g. dehydration, electrolyte imbalance, gallstones, heart and thyroid problems).

If you eat when you feel hungry, and opt for nutritious, whole foods that give your body sustained energy, your metabolism won't slow down. If you take your time while being thorough and implementing the strategies in this book, you will lose weight without ever regaining it. This is because you will not just go on a diet – you will embrace a new lifestyle.

Key Points and Strategies

- Acknowledge that you do have willpower or you wouldn't be able to make choices
- In a battle between hunger and willpower, hunger will always win
- Hunger is only desirable just before a meal
- Preventing yourself from getting hungry is your number one priority if you want to lose weight
- Keeping a food diary will make you aware of everything you eat
- Recognise your hunger, assess its intensity and record it in your diary
- Always eat when you're hungry, and stop eating when you're full • Fill up on complex carbohydrates and fibre to keep hunger at bay
- Include a serve of lean protein with each meal to help you feel satisfied
- Slow down your eating: after food enters your mouth, it takes about 20 minutes for the brain to realise that you're filling up
- Eat more vegetables
- Eat one-course meals to control your appetite

- Five or six small meals may work better than three big ones
- Plan your meals in advance
- Allow some flexibility with mealtimes according to your hunger feelings, but prepare a nutritious snack if you need to skip a meal
- Remember that you can eat tomorrow what you can't eat today
- Practice self-discipline by saying no to calorie-dense foods
- Do something you enjoy when you're tempted to eat for reasons other than genuine hunger.

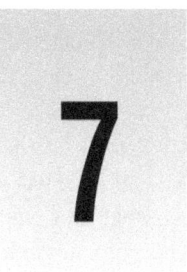

7

MOTIVATION: THE CORNERSTONE OF SUCCESS

Make a decision to be motivated, and keep your motivation alive.

Motivation comes from feeling good, and you feel good when you're the captain of own your ship. Directing your own life gives you a feeling of empowerment, and your diet is an essential part of this process. You control how you nourish your body. You can choose one course of action over another, while knowing what is best for you. You can choose meals and snacks that have all the nutrients your body requires, without creating a calorie surplus.

Motivation is an inner engine that keeps you going, even though it may not always be constant. Sometimes it is very strong and you find that losing weight is the easiest thing in the world. At other times, it is as though your motivation has left you: you wonder where it is and if it will ever come back. Emotions are powerful motivators: you can be motivated by negative feelings such as fear, envy or even revenge. But much more powerful are positive feelings, which will give you the incentive you need to continue, in spite of difficulties and setbacks.

If you think you *have to* lose weight, you will probably procrastinate forever. You will say, 'I will start my diet tomorrow, so I might as well eat all I want today.' But tomorrow might never come, so you continue to eat excessively and put on more weight. Instead of thinking you *have* to do it, why not say you *choose* to do it because it is what you want. You want to do it because you look forward to the end result. Looking forward to something (joyful anticipation) is the best feeling when deciding to lose weight. You can look forward to being healthy, more youthful and more energetic.

Motivation is a desire to do something, a willingness to achieve your goal. But the desire alone is not enough; action needs to follow. Use your intelligence to plan what you will do to get from A to B. This is *your* journey, and the best way to arrive at your desired destination is to make it as enjoyable as possible. Begin by setting things into motion to overcome inertia. Take a small step to get started. Empty your kitchen of high calorie items such as chocolate bars, cookies and potato chips – no, I don't mean eat it! – and replace them with wholesome foods such as fruit, vegetables, wholemeal pasta, plain yoghourt and lean chicken or fish.

If this step seems too drastic and you're not ready for it, do something less threatening. Research healthy eating and find as many recipes as you can. Collect them for later and think about what kind of meals you would like to eat. Design meal plans to suit your lifestyle. Say to yourself: 'I'm going to eat healthy today only. I will start with a good breakfast of unsweetened porridge and fruit. I will have nutritious snacks ready to take with me to work. I will stick to this plan for today only and see how I feel.'

You might enjoy it so much that you will want to do it again the next day, and the next! One day at a time is less daunting than having to do it for the rest of your life. Focus on getting started, without worrying about whether you will achieve your goal, how and when. Don't be a perfectionist, as this will put you under too much pressure. If you make mistakes, accept them and forgive yourself straight away, without punishing yourself. The occasional ice cream won't ruin your diet if you're sensible most of the time.

It takes courage to change, and obstacles will be in your way: fear, doubt and insecurity. Inner resistance can be overcome if you decide not to pay attention to it. Perhaps there is proof that you have failed in the past, and will fail again in the future, but why dwell on discouraging thoughts? Refuse to look at negative evidence. Keep the picture of your success in your mind, and see yourself the way you would like to be. Imagine what it would feel like, and cling to this feeling, no matter what. The past won't propel you forward; only the vision of good things to come will push you along. Even if you do nothing and keep reading this book over and over, you will begin to change. You will begin to lose weight, almost magically, as your new awareness will transform you.

Losing weight takes a long time. It's a process that can stretch over several months, sometimes even years. As you progress along the way, you will perceive a positive change in your attitude towards food and towards yourself. But this change doesn't happen overnight. It's the result of days, weeks and months of positive feedback from a new diet and lifestyle. Acknowledge what this diet is doing for you and feel grateful for it. If you find reasons to be thankful, it will be easier for you to stay on the right track. It will be effortless, instead of being a struggle.

Write down some positive aspects of your weight loss program. How do you benefit from it, even though you may not have lost a huge amount of weight yet? For example:

- I feel better already
- I feel lighter and move around more easily
- I sleep better and wake up refreshed in the morning
- I feel less bloated
- My ankles don't swell up any more
- I don't have so many aches and pains
- My eyes are brighter and my complexion is clearer
- My mood and my self-esteem have improved
- It makes me feel good to take care of myself and eat healthy
- I don't crave junk food so much
- I spend less money on processed and packaged foods
- My partner and/or my children enjoy the nutritious meals I prepare
- I never knew I loved vegetables so much
- I never knew there were so many different ways to prepare them.

The strategy of keeping your long-term goal in mind to stay motivated might not always work. Long-term goals can seem abstract and out of reach. You may cling to an idea or an ideal, but if it seems too far away or unrealistic, it won't spur you on effectively. You need something more concrete, something you can acknowledge *now* rather than in six months' time. If you feel your resolve weakening, don't just focus on the long-term benefits of your weight loss program. Think about the immediate benefits of a healthy diet and exercise program.

The Benefits of exercise are numerous, even in the absence of weight loss:

- **Improved insulin sensitivity.** More glucose enters your body cells, and your blood sugar level remains constant. As a result, you're less inclined to overeat. You feel less hungry, which may seem like a paradox, as you may feel hungry after a workout. But overall, your appetite and cravings diminish after exercising, and this effect lasts 24 hours.
- **Better mood.** You feel more relaxed, more optimistic and more energetic, due to an increase in the brain of serotonin and dopamine.
- **Lower blood pressure.** Start slow, by incorporating some physical activity into your daily routine. Regular exercise makes your heart stronger, and a stronger heart is able to pump blood more effectively. As your heart works less strenuously, the force on your arteries diminishes, and your blood pressure decreases. Exercise also makes your arteries more elastic, which further lowers your blood pressure, as your arteries offer less resistance to blood flow.
- **Improved bowel motility.** Exercise stimulates intestinal activity and helps prevent constipation. This beneficial effect is amplified by a diet high in fibre.
- **Better sleep.** Exercise helps you sleep more soundly at night, especially if you do it on a regular basis. You wake up more alert and more enthusiastic.

You can keep your motivation alive by focusing on the *process* rather than the end-result. The journey is as important as the destination. You may enjoy it so much that you will remember it as a positive and enlightening period of your life. Even though you may encounter numerous obstacles, you will remember the feeling of exhilaration as you progress on your path to health.

Every hurdle you overcome is a learning opportunity you can incorporate into your experience. Write your own list of immediate benefits, *how* and *why* your diet is making you feel better. This will inspire you and stop you from becoming disheartened as you encounter difficulties, like a seemingly never-ending plateau.

When she started out on her weight loss journey, Anna, 36, found that a calendar and a diary were valuable tools to keep on track. She wanted to lose weight to have more energy. Tiredness had always been a problem for her; at one stage she even thought she suffered from chronic fatigue syndrome. But the real culprit was her excess weight: it was robbing her of her vitality. She had to be honest and accept herself with all her strengths and weaknesses. She knew she could never completely give up chocolate. She had to cultivate motivation like a delicate plant. Her progress was encouraging, even though it was a bit slow during times when she hit a plateau. By keeping track of her weight loss on a chart, she could see that she was moving closer to her goal. She looked at this diagram whenever she felt depressed or fed up.

Acknowledging your achievements is an incentive for you to continue. A piece of written evidence can be a powerful nudge in the right direction. Having photos of yourself taken at regular intervals can also remind you that you *are* making progress. Stick them on the fridge, and look at them whenever you get tempted to deviate from your eating plan. A private online photo album is a good idea if you don't want anyone to see these pictures.

It may be difficult to get started, and the amount of weight you need to lose may seem overwhelming. I advise readers to divide the task ahead into small, manageable steps and focus on one baby step at a time. With your weight loss goal in mind, you can commit yourself to losing one kilogram a month. Start with the first month and look forward to the result, without worrying about what will happen afterwards.

By preparing yourself mentally *before* you change your eating habits, you will have a better chance to succeed, and you will avoid 'falling off the wagon'. Be clear about *why* you need to change: list all your reasons, even if they seem frivolous (e.g.: I want to wear fashionable clothes).

Follow a plan that suits your ideas and lifestyle. Design a schedule for shopping, as you will need fresh food on a regular basis, especially fruit and vegetables. If you've survived on ready meals and takeaways so far, your kitchen might lack basic equipment, so make sure you have all the cooking implements you need; e.g. sauce pans, chopping board, blender, knives, sealable containers, salad bowl. Allow yourself some exercise time, either in the morning before work, or in the evening after work. If you can't exercise every day, commit yourself to doing it at least two or three times a week.

Keeping a food diary is one of the most powerful tools for weight loss, as it makes you aware of everything you eat throughout the day. Once you keep a diary and you're completely honest, you can't live in denial any more. Everything has to be written down, every sweet or salty snack and every sugary drink. You can also use this diary to record physical activity, whether it's intense or just a stroll in the park. Any kind of exercise will make a difference, but, if you haven't done it in a long time, running a marathon is not indicated. If in doubt, consult your doctor first.

Once you're ready, set a *starting date* for your diet and exercise plan. Reward yourself once you've eaten healthily for a week (e.g. buy yourself a book, treat yourself to a massage or a facial). Plan ahead for treats: everyone enjoys an ice-cream once in a while, and including it in your plan will stop you from craving it.

Before you embark on your journey, picture all the possible scenarios that you will be confronted with that may lead you to be tempted. If you become aware of the process that leads you to give in to these urges, you will be able to overcome them. And if you've already given in, it's not too late to stop yourself. You may have opened the packet of crisps, but it doesn't mean you have to eat them.

You have a choice, every time you are about to put something in your mouth. You choose to be healthy and lead a productive and rewarding life, because you love yourself enough to give yourself this opportunity. Once you know what you want and *why* you want it, you won't have to go to war against yourself any more. The struggle will end, because you're following your true desire to be healthy, rather than giving in to the short-lived promise of instant gratification.

Don't be overwhelmed by the amount of work you need to do to lose weight. 'The best thing about the future is that it comes one day at a time,' said Abraham Lincoln. And the best way to deal with losing weight is to do it just for today. Don't look too far ahead, or you'll get worried and anxious. Focus on the *now*. Focus on the next step: the kilogram you've decided to lose this month. Success is like a staircase: you climb it one step at a time. To make a house, you lay the first brick, then the second, the third, and so on.

Everything you do adds up: every little step, every tiny effort to change your eating and exercise habits. With time and practice, you will find it easier to eat a healthy diet. At first you may need a lot of willpower, but after a while your actions will become automatic. You will adopt good habits and you won't need bucketloads of willpower. Patience is the key to lasting results, as you continue despite difficulties and setbacks. Discouragement may set in, but you don't allow it to influence your decision. You go on in spite of it.

Accept that you will make mistakes: if you very likely overeat from time to time, so don't see it as a failure. Mistakes are great learning opportunities, and how you deal with them makes the difference between giving up and persevering. People abandon their diet because they find it too hard. They want to do it by the book, or not at all. They don't allow themselves any flexibility. This all or nothing attitude is detrimental, as you'll end up punishing yourself and eating even more.

'I broke my diet, so I might as well eat as much as possible today, and start afresh tomorrow. I made mistakes today, so there is no guarantee that I won't make even more tomorrow. I can't follow this stupid diet – I'll fail again and succumb to binging.'

This kind of thinking is harmful and counter-productive, because it won't lead you anywhere. It's also depressing. To fail over and over is not motivating. Erase the concept of failure from your mind once and for all. There is no such thing!

You're on a journey, and losing weight is a process. It takes time to change and to make adjustments. It's all about learning, and you can never fail if you look at it this way. You may have eaten too much or indulged in calorie-laden food on one occasion, but your next meal can be a healthy one. This kind of thinking is the only way to get back on track. Look at the big picture and at your overall progress, rather than concentrating on isolated events and actions. Motivation is not always steady: it can be strong one day and weak, almost inexistent the next. Accept that you can't be perfect and you won't be so hard on yourself!

This book is not a diet in the traditional sense. You don't have to stick to it religiously. There are no commands, just suggestions to help you improve your wellbeing and body shape. It's about freedom, choice and responsibility. It's not just about the food you consume and how many kilograms show up on the scales. The transformation you'll experience is internal: in your mind as well as your body. It is long-lasting because it's a change of attitude towards food and yourself. You don't have to feel guilty any more. Instead of beating up on yourself, you accept yourself and forgive yourself. You *use* your mistakes to expand your knowledge and experience. This is how you get to know yourself better.

Feeling guilt and shame about a binge or other misstep won't help. Remind yourself that there is nothing you can do to change the *past*. Worrying about the future won't help you either. You only have today – so stop saying 'Tomorrow, I'm going on a diet.' Instead, you could say to yourself:

'From This *moment* on, I will eat a healthy diet, starting now, one day at a time. I will trust myself that I can do it. Every time I am about to eat, I am conscious that I have a choice. I don't have to be perfect. If I overeat, I won't punish myself. Instead, I will learn from it and I will be good to myself. I will treat myself with compassion and understanding, while encouraging myself to stay on the path I've chosen for myself.'

Every day, you have the opportunity to choose what you will eat and how much of it. Just cutting down on your eating and portion sizes can work wonders. Using a small plate and filling it up may be good to control portions, as the same amount of food can look larger on a small plate. But spreading your food on a big plate can also make it look like *more,* rather than cramming it on a tiny plate. See what works best for you, as you eat with your eyes just as you eat with your mouth.

Losing weight is being aware of choices and alternatives. Instead of eating biscuits to fill a void, you could eat fruit. I never used to believe that fruit could be enough to satisfy hunger between meals, until I tried it, and it worked! You don't have to be perfect at everything you're doing. Do something just because you want to do it, without any expectations, and you will lose weight.

Key Points and Strategies:

- Use positive thoughts to motivate yourself
- Be aware of *why* you want to lose weight
- Write a list of things you're grateful for *now*, thanks to your new eating habit
- Use a good system to monitor your progress, and reward yourself for your achievements
- Set yourself short-term goals and lose weight little by little
- Only lose one kilogram at a time: one kilogram a month is a sensible target
- Stop being a perfectionist: mistakes are normal, and they are important learning opportunities
- Stop punishing yourself. Forgive yourself right away and don't dwell on your mistakes
- Banish guilt, 'the useless emotion': it does nothing for you, and it stops you from achieving your goal
- Replace guilt with *trust* in yourself and the knowledge that you can do it
- Eat a healthy diet, one day at a time
- Realise you have a choice, every time you're about to put something in your mouth.

8

WHAT CAN YOU EAT?

It's not how much you eat, but what you eat that makes the difference.

If you were only indulging too freely in wholemeal bread, grains, cereals, pasta, sweet potatoes, fresh fruit and vegetables, as well as lean protein such as fish, prawns or chicken breast, chances are you would be lean and fit rather than fat. Overeating is not always a problem, unless you eat a lot of unhealthy, fattening food! People don't binge on fruit and vegetables, and it seems that overeating is linked to junk foods and fast food restaurants, as well as processed foods and grocery retailers. The problem is not so much the volume, but the *type* of food you eat.

Your day-to-day choices determine your state of health, but you can only make these choices if you have the necessary information or knowledge. This book will guide you in the direction of healthy choices, as you gain a better understanding about food and what it does to you. You will understand what role carbohydrates, protein and fat play in your body. You will understand why it's important to eat fresh foods high in fibre.

If you were stranded on an island in the middle of the ocean, with only fresh food available like fish, coconut and tropical fruit, no television, no internet and no car, you would end up losing weight, even if you didn't intend to do so. The healthy lifestyle you would be compelled to adopt would make you slim down the natural way. But you live in a complex, high-tech society where highly processed foods are a reality you can never completely avoid. You can only try to keep them to a minimum. Be aware that, day after day, your food choices determine your health and waistline.

There are five popular diet myths that will mislead people and encourage them to fail at dieting:

1) You must avoid sugar at all cost. While it is true that excessive sugar can be harmful, cutting it out altogether is not necessary. You can still enjoy your favourite treats and desserts in moderation, as a part of a healthy meal plan. Refined sugar is one of the things we enjoy as human beings, so telling you that you will never be able to eat it any more is unrealistic. Instead of saying, 'Never eat sugar', I prefer to say, 'Eat sugar sensibly'. Reduce it to a minimum but enjoy it consciously. Savour every morsel of cake, and suck on a piece of chocolate instead of crunching it.

2) A high protein diet is best. Too much protein can be harmful. Low carbohydrate diets are no better, as they are high protein diets in disguise. The world famous Dr Atkins was the first to promote this type of weight loss regimen, which admittedly works to some degree, at least in the beginning. While it looks attractive, because you can consume as much protein and fat as you like, it is detrimental as it causes ketosis, a chemical imbalance that occurs when your body burns fat in the absence of carbohydrates. This may sound good, but it is unpleasant and even dangerous. The signs are bad breath, weakness, headache, tiredness, dizziness, anxiety, insomnia and nausea and constipation.

By cutting out carbohydrates you become serotonin deprived, and this will lead to low energy, low mood and food cravings. Looming around the corner is a big carbohydrate binge! Long-term effects of the Atkins diet are high cholesterol, heart disease, premature aging, osteoporosis and cancer. There is also a rebound effect: you will put on even more weight when you revert to eating carbohydrates.

3) You must reduce carbohydrates drastically. Rather than eliminating something, or reducing it to a minimum, a better alternative is to simply eat a balanced diet. Focus on whole grain products, pulses and vegetables, as they are a good source of fibre and will be digested slowly, keeping your blood sugar levels more even.

4) You must eat a fat-free diet. In the 1980s, dietary recommendations encouraged everyone to adopt low-fat diets. This advice did more damage than good, and is probably responsible for an increase in weight gain and obesity. Fats are beneficial and an important part of a balanced eating plan. While it is sensible to *moderate* your fat intake, going without or with too little of this essential nutrient is counterproductive. Fat suppresses ghrelin, the hormone that makes you feel hungry, while simultaneously spurring the release of peptides that make you feel full.

Saturated fats found in meats and dairy products are beneficial, as they are sources of important nutrients and help absorb essential fatty acids, fat-soluble vitamins, and calcium. Avoid trans-fatty acids found in fast foods and processed foods such as biscuits, ready-made pies and cakes, pizzas, potato chips, doughnuts, confectionery and dessert mixes. These trans fats are harmful because they cause nutritional deficiencies, especially in essential omega 3 and omega 6 fatty acids, which are needed to build healthy cells and maintain brain and nerve function in the body. Vegetable oils (except for cold pressed coconut oil) can be harmful too, if consumed in excess or at high temperatures, as they release toxins that can damage your body cells.

5) All you need to do is restrict your caloric intake. This approach may sound effective, if you consider that excessive calories are the origin of weight gain; to address this problem you need to create a caloric deficit by burning more calories than you consume. In theory this may work, but in practice, it's not enough.

You may still eat the wrong kind of food and become vitamin and mineral deficient. You may not consume enough fibre, and choose refined products such as polished rice or white pasta. You may consume low quality protein such as sausages or patties. You may end up not only malnourished, but literally *starving*, as you won't have enough nutrients in your diet. A calorie-restrictive diet could be risky, and hunger could take over, disempowering you and leading you to break your diet. It can also slow your metabolism as your body goes into starvation mode.

Instead of focusing on what you can't eat, focus on what you *can* eat. Choose a variety of nutritious foods out of the following groups:

1 - GRAINS AND LEGUMES (rich in complex carbohydrates): five to seven serves or more a day, according to age and level of activity (one serve = one slice of bread, one medium potato, half a cup of cooked oats, brown rice or whole meal pasta).

Have oats (a bowl of porridge with fruit is a good way to start the day), wholemeal bread and pasta, brown rice, potatoes, legumes such as lentils, peas, beans or chick peas. Legumes need to be soaked overnight, drained and cooked, but you can buy them canned or pre-cooked for convenience.

2 - FRUIT AND VEGETABLES: five to seven serves or more (one serve = one piece of fruit, one cup of diced or canned fruit, half a cup of cooked vegetables, half a cup of corn kernels, one cup of salad vegetables). Preferably, fruit and vegetables should be eaten raw or lightly cooked (except in soups) but for convenience you may occasionally use canned or frozen veggies.

3 - LEAN BEEF, FISH, SEAFOOD, CHICKEN (SKINLESS), TOFU, NUTS OR EGGS: two to three serves a day (one serve = 100g of lean meat, fish, chicken, tofu, two large eggs; 30g of nuts, peanut or almond butter).

Dietary cholesterol used to be considered a major cause of unhealthy blood cholesterol, and egg yolks have been wrongly demonized ever since. You may have been told to eat egg whites only. While egg whites may be great, especially when you're cooking a dish that requires a lot of eggs, whole eggs should be included in a healthy diet. You can definitely have your egg and eat the yolk too!

Dietary cholesterol is not the true villain. Some studies have found that egg yolk helps reduce LDL ('bad' cholesterol). Egg yolk is full of omega-3 fatty acids, B vitamins, protein and other valuable nutrients.

Lean meat, poultry, fish and egg are not the only foods rich in protein. Legumes, as well as seeds and nuts such as almonds (one serve (= ¼ cup) can replace a meat serve if you're a vegan. They are also important sources of protein, while providing fibre, which meat does not.

4 - MILK, DAIRY PRODUCTS OR SOY MILK: two or three serves, four if you're a woman and over 50 (one serve: 250 ml low fat milk, 200 g plain, low fat, unsweetened yoghourt, a quarter of a cup of cottage cheese, 40 g of hard cheese or soy cheese).

5 – BUTTER, OLIVE OIL OR COCONUT OIL: two or three teaspoons at the most.

6 - OCCASIONAL INDULGENCE: once or twice a week, treat yourself to something you enjoy, but in moderation: two or three slices of salami, a square of chocolate, a handful of chips or crisps, one or two cream biscuits, small piece of cake, small glass of fruit juice or 'slushy'.

Note: Serves and quantities are suggestions only. They follow the Australian dietary guidelines: 'Eat for Health' .Variations are allowed and encouraged according to height and genetics, age, sex, and level of activity. A professional athlete or dancer requires more daily calories than a labourer, who in turn needs more than an office worker. If you're unsure about what and how much you should eat according to your body type, circumstances and any possible medical condition, please consult a dietician or nutritionist for an individualized diet plan.

Be aware that anything too high in fat or sugar can contribute to weight gain, if you eat it too often or in large quantities. Make it your responsibility to find out about the nutritional value of the food you eat. You don't need to turn into a mathematician; allow your common sense to guide you. The science of weight loss is not the science of deprivation; it's the science of choices. The greater your knowledge, the more effective your choices will be. By choosing low fat spinach bake instead of cheese cake, you're making progress towards your goal.

Take time to enjoy your food. A lot of overweight people tend to eat on the run, never sitting down to have proper meals. Take time to *relax* while eating, and make yourself as comfortable as possible. Avoid all distractions: TV, internet, social media. Turn off your phone if you're tempted to text.

Mealtimes should be special times. In a lot of cultures, purifying rituals are performed before meals and a lot of Christians say grace. To put you in the right frame of mind and stop you from rushing through your meal while thinking about something else, allow yourself to focus on what you're eating. Reflect on the food which is a gift, and there to satisfy your hunger and to be enjoyed.

Chew every morsel thoroughly while concentrating on what you're putting in your mouth. Focus on taste, texture and consistency, and how food travels to your stomach. Chewing gives your brain more time to process information and to receive the message of satiety. The more you chew, the fuller you feel, and the less you're likely to overeat!

Key Points and Strategies:

- Don't adhere to a drastic food regimen
- Don't go on a high protein or a low carbohydrate diet
- Don't cut fat too low, but use healthy fats
- Cholesterol is not the culprit, and egg yolks are okay
- Choose healthy foods whenever you can
- Allow yourself the occasional indulgence, but in moderation
- Take time to enjoy your food
- Sit down for your meals
- Make yourself comfortable and relax
- Avoid distractions and turn off technology
- Chew your food thoroughly
- Take time to taste your food and to be grateful for it.

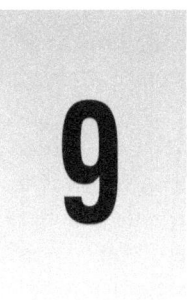

9

FAT AND 'TOXIC WASTE'

Detoxify your body and your fat will disappear.

Jerry, 41, married with three children, weighs 140 kilograms. An earthmoving contractor and the owner of two loaders and a truck, he has always been a big-framed person, but he is now more overweight than he's ever been.

Jerry works ten hours a day, six days a week. On his way to work, he has a ham and cheese croissant and muffins with a tall latte. For lunch, he has either pies with sauce, hotdogs or hamburgers with hot chips and he drinks half a litre of Coke (not the sugar-free version). He has jam doughnuts and cream buns for afternoon tea with iced coffee.

Jerry never eats fruit or vegetables (he calls it 'rabbit food'), apart from a few overcooked peas or carrots that he wife makes him eat with his dinner, which usually consists of a big piece of meat (pork or beef), mashed potatoes, rich gravy and pork crackling. As well as smoking a packet of cigarettes a day and drinking six cans of beer after work, he takes a lot of Panadol and Nurofen, as he suffers from headaches and a bad back.

Jerry is worried about his health, which is deteriorating. Last time he went to see his doctor, he was told that he had high cholesterol, high blood pressure, that his liver enzymes were up and that he was a borderline diabetic. He was told that if he didn't lose weight and change his lifestyle, he would have a heart attack or a stroke, or develop full-blown diabetes.

Jerry doesn't believe that he can do it, because his previous attempts at losing weight failed, and he's not sure how to go about it. But the other day, his mechanic said to him: 'If you didn't put so much rubbish into your body, you would lose weight.' This sentence struck him and he suspects there is some truth in it.

An Australian bestseller for almost twenty years, 'The Liver Cleansing Diet: Love your Liver and Live Longer' by Dr Sandra Cabot is still one of the best weight loss guides, due to its common-sense approach. Using illustrations and funny cartoons, it explains how the liver works and the importance of keeping this organ healthy.

Dr Cabot presents a detailed eight-week plan to promote vitality and longevity by cleansing your liver. The book follows basics like eliminating processed foods, alcohol, sugar, and too much saturated fat from dairy products and red meat. Some saturated fat is okay as part of a healthy diet and moderation is the key. The bulk of your diet should consist of fresh vegetables, fruit, fish, whole grains, free range chicken, and lots of fibre.

Avoid cooking in fat and use water instead, sprinkling cold pressed olive oil just before the end of the process. Heating up fats changes their shape, and they become trans-fats. These are also the fats found in processed foods (the kind that Jerry loves to eat on a daily basis).

The liver has a hard time processing them and it becomes clogged up with them, which affects its ability to remove toxins from the blood, as well a manufacturing and storing important substances. The liver produces bile, a greenish substance which emulsifies fats in your bowels. It stores iron and certain vitamins, produces amino acids essential for survival, as well as hormones.

The liver plays an essential role in your carbohydrate metabolism by making, storing and releasing glucose at appropriate times. It also has several roles in the metabolism of fat. It makes cholesterol which is essential for hormone and bile production. The liver also produces coagulation factors; this is why excessive bleeding can be a sign of liver dysfunction.

The liver breaks down toxic substances, turning them into harmless metabolites that the body can easily eliminate. It also breaks down medicines, like the Panadol that Jerry takes, by a process called drug metabolisms. When your liver doesn't work properly, toxins accumulate in your body and can lead to serious health complaints. They can also be the origin of allergies and auto-immune diseases.

You liver is bigger than your brain, and it is your major fat burning organ. It is a *detoxification* organ, but, if it is constantly overworked and clogged up with fats and toxins, it will not be able to perform its duties properly. The first thing that will suffer is your *metabolism,* which will slow down as much as possible, so the liver can catch up on other, more important things. Fats will not be broken down properly, and will accumulate in your abdominal area, producing the 'pot belly' or 'muffin top'.

When your liver functions properly, it burns all excess calories instead of storing them as fat. If you want to enjoy the benefits of an effective fat-burning machine, make sure you eat the foods I recommend in this book. They match Dr Cabot's recommendations, apart from a few variations: I won't ask you to eliminate dairy products, unless you wish to do so. Iron supplements may be advisable for women who consume little or no red meat.

Fibre is essential for good liver function, as it mops up excess bile and fats in your bowels during digestion. If your liver is overworked, it won't produce sufficient bile, and if you don't eat enough fibre (as in Jerry's case), part of the bile that reaches your bowels will be reabsorbed and recycled, resulting in high levels of LDL, the 'bad' cholesterol. Your arteries will be coated with calcified fat deposits that will harden and narrow them, which eventually will push your blood pressure up to dangerous levels. Once a blood vessel is completely obstructed, you'll end up with a heart attack (due to a blocked coronary artery) or a stroke (due to a blocked blood vessel in your brain)

Body fat can be used by the liver to store substances that it is not able to process at the moment. These toxins are put aside to be dealt with later. Fat has an active role as the liver's 'helper' and rather than being the sluggish, inert mass we once thought it was, it has a very active role. The body will resist losing fat if the liver doesn't function adequately. If all your excess fat were burnt at once, there would be an overload of accumulated toxins invading your bloodstream, and this could be lethal. The more overweight you are, the wiser it is to lose weight slowly and steadily, allowing your liver to recover and regenerate itself so it can go on burning fat effectively.

Body fat protects your body from toxins. Besides chemicals in your diet and medicines, many of the foods you eat (especially items like packaged and manufactured foods, fizzy drinks, biscuits, ice creams, chips and confectionary, which are usually loaded with sugar, salt and trans fats) produce 'toxic waste'. Your body is like a factory: everything you ingest has to be metabolized: *transformed* to be used for your needs. At the same time, your body has to get rid of all the 'rubbish' resulting in the process.

Your liver and kidneys are constantly busy removing wasteful products from your body. If you consistently overeat, and ingest a lot of junk food as well as other poisons like nicotine or alcohol, you'll overload your system with toxins your liver and kidneys won't be able to eliminate any more. Your body will store these toxins as fat, which is a protective mechanism as it stops them from causing havoc. Your body stores the poisons it can't cope with in your fat cells.

Going on a restrictive diet can be dangerous. Fat stores break down too fast, releasing excessive amounts of harmful substances into your bloodstream. A horror scenario for your overworked liver! Crash diets literally cause a kind of blood poisoning. The symptoms are anxiety, panic attacks, nervousness, sleeplessness, fatigue and strong cravings for processed foods full of sugar, salt and fat. Your instinct tells you to eat fattening foods, so you can quickly replenish your fat store and feel normal again.

Besides sugar, salt and trans-fats, processed foods often contain harmful chemicals: colourings, preservatives, artificial flavours, acidity regulators, anti-caking, anti-foaming or glazing agents, emulsifiers, stabilizers, thickeners or bulking agents. Fruit and vegetables contain pesticides and our drinking water is not free of chemicals from industrial waste. You can't avoid chemicals entirely. Even the ocean contains pollutants that affect fish and seafood.

You could become self-sufficient and only eat from your organic vegetable garden. But even then, acid rain, ground and water pollution could still affect you. All you can do is avoid highly processed foods, which are full of chemicals. Choose organic or free range products whenever possible and if your budget allows it. It's better to eat non-organic vegetables than not eat any vegetables at all!

Fruit, vegetables, beans, seeds, nuts and whole grains will help you detoxify your body. Carrot, cabbage, Brussels sprouts, apple, grapefruit, beetroot, garlic, avocado, banana, leafy greens and green tea are particularly good for your liver. Moderate exercise might not burn many calories, but it activates the cleansing process by stimulating your liver and kidneys, helping them to rid the body of toxins. Sweating is an effective way to carry waste out of the system.

People take prescription drugs to treat symptoms that wouldn't be there if they changed their lifestyle. High blood pressure, high cholesterol, and even diabetes in its early stages can be reversed by modifying your diet and lifestyle. In *The Magic of Willpower*, I explain how to change your habits by replacing them with new ones. After a while, your new habit becomes automatic. It requires less willpower, as it has become a part of you, and you feel awkward without it. When you don't brush your teeth, you don't feel right. Because you do it every day, you miss it if you fail to do it.

If you're serious about losing weight, you can't simply cut down on food. Consider everything you put into your body, and ask yourself if you really need it. Pharmaceuticals in particular should only be taken if absolutely necessary, and in the lowest possible dose. We live in an age of instant gratification, and expect doctors to remove bothersome symptoms right away. We expect to leave the surgery with at least a script in our hands.

Be grateful if your doctor doesn't give you a script. Shop around for a doctor who takes time to *listen* to you and doesn't treat you like a number. Your doctor should be empathetic, non-judgmental and open to natural treatments alongside traditional ones. A script can be a cop out. Sensible advice on how to change your lifestyle and regain your health would be more helpful and effective in the long run.

Every drug has side effects, so make an informed decision before taking any medication. Inform yourself about the possible negative effects. Even the ubiquitous paracetamol (acetaminophen in the U.S.A.), wrongly believed to be harmless, is toxic and can cause irreversible liver damage. Paracetamol toxicity is the most common cause of acute liver failure in the Western world, and accounts for most drug overdoses in the United States, the United Kingdom, Australia and New Zealand.

All drugs are chemicals that don't belong in your body and may potentially harm you. Complaints like nervousness, sleeplessness, constipation or heartburn can be relieved with drugs, but there are gentler ways to address them. Better food, more water, more rest, relaxation, gentle exercise, meditation and even prayer can do wonders. In the long run, drugs may worsen your condition. Valium (diazepam), for instance, is often prescribed to treat anxiety, but one of its long-term side effects *is* anxiety.

Serious conditions such as cancer, pneumonia or major depression require chemical drugs, but it's always a good idea to seek a second or third opinion, especially if you're unhappy with the amount or type of drugs you have to take. Avoid taking over-the-counter products like cold and flu tablets, laxatives and painkillers. No one should endure chronic, disabling pain, but avoid taking a tablet for every little ache. Give your headache a chance to go away on its own before taking anything for it.

Even herbal remedies are not always innocuous, so check with a doctor or naturopath before using them. I believe that vitamin C and garlic are harmless remedies for common colds and other infections. They can boost your immune system and help your body fight off invading agents. Young children in particular seem to benefit from vitamin C. As a mother, I often found it to be more powerful than antibiotics to cure my children of minor ailments like sore throats, runny noses and coughs. Vitamin C is also helpful to reduce allergies, as it is a mild antihistamine.

Eat a healthy diet, and reduce the amount of chemicals you ingest. Lose weight as *slowly* as possible. As your fat burns little by little, it will only release negligible amounts of poison into your bloodstream. Don't go on a crash diet and lose weight too quickly, as you will pay the price for it. Your liver and kidneys will be overworked; toxins will remain in your blood and make you sick. This is why you feel unwell when you lose weight quickly: you're actually poisoning yourself!

You can lose weight permanently if you love your body *and* your liver. Loving yourself is a good starting point. Accept your body as it is. Love your fat, so you can let go of it. If you're happy and you love yourself, you won't put harmful substances into your body. If you want to look after yourself, you will eat more fruit and vegetables, while avoiding pizzas, beer and cheese cakes.

The more you get to know your body and accept it, and love it the way it is (because it's the only one you've got), the more you will want to take care of yourself and adopt a healthy lifestyle. You will automatically reduce the amount of harmful foods and poisons you ingest. Your liver will recover and regenerate itself. It will become the fat-burning machine that it is meant to be.

The less 'rubbish' you put into your body, the less likely you will be to store fat. Fat becomes unnecessary in a 'clean' body. Slowly, all the toxins that have accumulated in your body over time will be washed away, and your fat will melt like snow in the sun.

Key Points and Strategies:

- If you want to lose weight and live longer, look after your liver
- Clean your liver by following the dietary principles in this book, or follow the Australian guidelines for healthy eating
- Avoid processed and take-away foods
- Avoid nicotine, alcohol and unnecessary pharmaceuticals
- Consume animal fat from meat and dairy in moderation
- Avoid cooking and frying in fat
- Avoid trans-fats, salt and sugar
- Prevent your body from storing poisons as fat
- Eat raw fruit and vegetables, especially carrot, cabbage, Brussels sprouts, apple, grapefruit, beetroot, garlic, avocado, banana and leafy greens
- Drink green tea without milk or sugar
- Eat beans, seeds, nuts and whole grains
- Exercise moderately to detoxify your body
- Lose weight *slowly t*o avoid 'blood poisoning' and rebound weight gain
- If you really love your body you won't put rubbish into it.

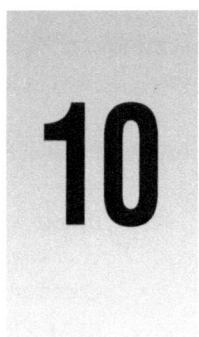

10

CALORIE-COUNTING IS
COUNTER-PRODUCTIVE

Lose weight without counting calories.

Sandra, 48, Clinical Nurse Manager in an aged care facility, didn't want to go on a diet. She hated the idea of counting calories. She couldn't picture herself weighing every single item, and doing the maths to work out the calories. It felt like going back to school and doing her homework.

Being an individualist, Sandra felt reluctant to submit to this kind of external control. Although Sandra was prepared to follow sensible guidelines for her diet, she didn't want to be told the exact number of calories she could eat per day. She found it too restrictive and frightening. And she feared that, if she started living that way, she would have to do it for the rest of her life.

What if she became obsessed with calorie-counting? What if she got it wrong? What if she ate more calories than the recommended amount? To her, this could easily mean ditching her diet or overindulging in high-calorie foods. Sandra wanted to feel in control of her food intake while having choices. She wanted freedom without the pressure to perform. Sandra should listen to her gut feeling, because calorie-counting can actually become a kind of eating disorder!

Calorie-counting can be helpful when you first reduce your food intake, especially if you've always had fairly large portions. Some people eat two or three times the recommended serving sizes, because they never measure their portions. You may have no idea what a regular food portion looks like. It may be helpful to weigh your food and count calories for a while, to give you an idea of what a healthy portion looks like.

Calorie-counting is a specific type of food diary. Food diaries have been proven to help with weight loss, as you keep yourself accountable for what you eat. It helps you realize how energy dense poor food choices are. A Big Mac burger meal with fries and a Coke has the energy equivalent of 70 % of the daily recommendation for sedentary women – without the fibre, vitamins, minerals and antioxidants found in fresh whole food. Hopefully, this awareness will encourage you to look for lower calorie - and healthier - options. Another advantage is that it will motivate you to work out regularly, although I believe it's the wrong approach to exercise, as it shouldn't be done with the sole intention of burning calories.

Excess weight is not caused by a lack of counting calories, just like sleeplessness is not caused by a lack of sleeping pills. Obesity, just like insomnia, is caused by something disturbing natural processes in the body, our innate regulatory systems. The most likely cause of obesity today is an excess of the fat-storing hormone *insulin*. This is the result of years of overindulging in sugar and highly processed, rapidly-digested carbohydrates as well as trans fats found in manufactured foods.

This type of eating, as well as the consumption of soft drinks (pop, fizzy drinks or soda), has messed up our hunger and satiety systems, making us want to eat excessively. Calorie-counting won't solve the problem. It's only a crutch, and the more you rely on it, the greater the chance of it turning into a neurotic activity that will take over your life. By counting calories, you learn *not* to rely on your body's instinctive ability to regulate your food intake. It's unnatural and ineffective in the long term.

Calorie-counting underestimates your natural ability to know when you're full. It's an artificial way to keep track of how much you're eating but, if you look into it properly, it doesn't make much sense. The idea behind it is to create a caloric deficit: if you consume less energy than your body requires, you will lose weight. But your body will adjust its metabolism according to the number of calories you put into it. If you eat a lot less than you need, your metabolism will slow down. If you eat slightly more, your metabolism will increase and burn excess energy, as long as your liver is working properly and you're reasonably active while eating healthy, nutritious food and a lot of fibre.

Calorie counting will put you under unnecessary pressure to hit your 'calorie goal'. If you exceed it, you will panic and possibly binge as a result. You will restrict your caloric intake even more, and your body will go into starvation mode. This is the body's natural response to a perceived threat when you don't eat enough calories. Your metabolism slows down, so your body can conserve energy to keep vital organs such as brain and heart functioning.

Along with fat, your body will start burning lean muscle for fuel, which will slow your metabolism even more. People on low calorie diets, especially 1000 calories a day and under, will invariably regain all the weight they've lost! High protein and low carbs diets have the same rebound effect, and after an initial period of success, they pave the way for more fat gain and resistance to weight loss.

A calorie is an artificial measurement that represents the amount of energy required to raise the temperature of one kilogram of water by one degree Centigrade. To confuse us even more, it is the norm nowadays to use kilojoules:

1 calorie (Cal) – 4.1868 kilojoules (kJ)

Calorie counting is not accurate. Researchers found that restaurant meals and dishes were found to have an average of 18 % more calories than stated. Frozen meals from supermarkets were found to contain an average of 8 % more. Some foods evaluated by scientists had more than twice as many calories as stated! This is scary when you realize that, theoretically, a caloric excess of just 5 % a day can cause five kilograms of weight gain in a single year! A low fat yoghourt that is supposed to have only 100 calories may in fact have 120 calories.

Cooked food also has more calories than raw food, and it takes more energy to digest protein than to digest fat or simple carbohydrates. The more muscle you have, the more calories you burn. The less you eat, the less calories you burn: your metabolism slows down, and your body may even use your lean muscles to produce energy.

According to Robert Lustig, MD, author of the book 'Fat Chance', the obesity epidemic is caused by the increase of sugar in our diet over the last decades, especially fructose. Fructose is added to about 80 % of processed supermarket shelf products. High fructose corn syrup tastes sweeter than sugar. It is used to make a lot of products more palatable, even those that don't normally contain sugar, like salad dressings or sauces. Sugar has 56 different names, which are used on packaging labels to confuse us.

To Robert Lustig, the problem is not obesity but metabolic syndrome. This cluster of symptoms is likely to lead to high cholesterol, high blood pressure, heart disease, type 2 diabetes, cancer and Alzheimer's disease. It is characterized by *visceral* fat: excess fat around your organs, which you may not even be aware of. Eating healthy is not just for the overweight or the obese, as you may be thin on the outside, but fat on the inside.

Robert Lustig explains that a calorie is NOT a calorie: calories from sugar are the worst kind of calories. Sugar is the culprit, and its excessive consumption has been directly linked to the obesity epidemic and metabolic syndrome. Robert Lustig proves that fructose is just as toxic as alcohol, as it is metabolized by the liver. Excessive fructose is turned into *fat* and accumulates in the liver, causing non-alcoholic fatty liver disease. It also gathers around major organs, while being stored in your fat cells.

Fructose is not dependent on insulin like regular sugar, but it leads to insulin resistance, as it indirectly causes the pancreas to release more insulin. Insulin stops the brain from recognizing *leptin,* which has disastrous consequences. Leptin is a substance that signals *fullness* and gives your body the message to become *active* and start releasing energy: you become more fidgety.

With insulin resistance, your body needs up to five times the normal amount of insulin to bring your blood glucose down to healthy levels. This in turn causes *hypoglycaemia* (low blood sugar) and a craving for more sugary foods. The pancreas produces even more insulin, which further blocks leptin signalling to your brain. As a result, you're always hungry, and you can't stop eating!

Leptin is an important hormone that regulates food intake and controls body weight. Fructose indirectly causes your brain to become *insensitive* to it, due to the overproduction of insulin that ensues. Fructose in itself does not cause hyperinsulinemia (too much insulin) but it leads to it indirectly.

Robert Lustig proves that sugar is a highly addictive substance. It stimulates *reward* centres in the brain, and its consumption is also linked to stress. Stress is a big problem in today's society. Youngsters, in particular, are vulnerable to all kinds of stressors due to school work, peer pressure and the Internet. To reverse sugar addiction it's important to stick to a wholesome diet of fresh foods, very low in sugar and high in fibre. This will regulate your insulin production and make your brain more sensitive to *leptin.* You will know when you're full, and when you've had enough to eat. And it has nothing to do with counting calories.

Counting calories or kilojoules is not recommended past the first couple of weeks of a new eating plan. Eat according to your natural hunger and satiety signals. These may not be obvious in the beginning, but as you consistently stick to a healthy diet, your brain will learn to recognize these signals. You will begin to be in tune with your body and its nutritional needs.

Over-consumption of sugar has desensitized you. By eliminating it from your diet and replacing it with fresh fruit, vegetables, whole grains, seeds, nuts and legumes, your body will recover. Counting calories is counter-productive: it can be harmful to drastically limit the amount of food you eat. It slows your metabolism and sets the stage for rebound weight gain. If you count calories, you'll probably end up carrying even more weight than you've lost.

Weight loss is not about mathematics, about adding or subtracting figures. Caloric energy alone is not responsible for your fat. Fat is a complex issue that can't be solved by a simple equation, or by creating a caloric deficit. A lot of people say they don't eat much, and they certainly don't lie. Their bodies have become resistant to burning fat, due to past crash diets and yoyo dieting.

Not all calories are the same. A calorie from refined sugar or fructose doesn't have the same effect as a calorie from complex carbohydrates. Eating a candy is not the equivalent of eating a banana, even if the caloric content is the same. Sugar tends to go straight to your fat stores and messes up your insulin production, while complex carbohydrates tend to be used as fuel during energy expenditure. In the long term, the same number of calories can produce either fat or energy.

Fibre absorbs excess fat in the digestive tract and in the bloodstream, and therefore acts like a calorie-saver, preventing these calories from being turned into more fat. Divide the same amount of calories into several small meals instead of three big ones, and you save even more calories by stimulating your metabolism. Calories you eat in the morning are less fattening than those you consume late at night. Whatever you eat in the early hours of the day will be used up as energy, but night-time eating will replenish your fat stores.

Because so many different parameters are involved, weight loss is not an accurate science. Many people find they can't stick to a diet, because the mental effort needed to measure portions of foods and count calories is too great. The good news is you don't have to do it! You're more likely to succeed if you *don't* count calories. Simply apply the principles in this book: your overall health and metabolism will improve, and you will lose weight gradually and naturally.

Some complicated equations can help you determine how many calories a day you should eat. But I don't believe it's useful, due to the many factors that can influence weight loss or gain. It's difficult to determine the energy needs of an individual from one day to the next. It makes more sense to *reduce* your portions sizes. Clasp your hands together in a ball. It will tell you how much you can eat, with the exception of fresh, preferably raw vegetables. You can eat as many vegetables as you like, as long as you don't add excessive amounts of butter, oil, dressing or other sauces to them.

Listen to your body: after a few weeks of healthy eating, it will tell you what it needs in order to thrive. Eating less won't shrink your stomach, contrary to popular belief, but it will reset your 'appetite thermostat': the intensity and frequency of your hunger is likely to decrease. Stretching your stomach with too much food is not a good idea: doing this on a regular basis will not help you stick to a weight loss plan! But if you cut calories below your comfort level, you will feel drained, nervous and fatigued, without stamina and without any desire to continue with your diet.

Make it you goal *never* to feel hungry, unless before a meal. If you still feel hungry after meals, add more complex carbohydrates to your diet, as they will give you the energy you need. Hunger is a natural body signal: listen to it, respect it and satisfy this need in a natural, wholesome way with the right kind of food.

Calorie counting puts you under pressure. It could lead you to eat foods you were trying to avoid. You become so desperate to break out of this 'jail' that overindulging seems the only way out, the only escape from a discipline that is too hard to cope with.

Be proactive and plan what you will eat from one day to the next, but don't be too restrictive and don't punish yourself. Calories are only numbers. You can make healthy food choices, knowing that your hunger and satiety feelings will guide you. This guidance system may not work right away, but it is guaranteed to kick in after a few weeks of healthy eating. Make a decision to *trust* your body, such a wonderful machine, perfectly designed in every way!

Key Points and Strategies:

1) Pros and cons of calorie-counting:

Pros:

- Counting calories may help you reduce your portion sizes
- You will keep a specific food diary that will make you accountable to yourself and others
- It may be an opportunity to learn more about healthy nutrition.

Cons:

- Calorie counting can lead to obsession and eating disorders; it's not recommended after the first two weeks
- A calorie is NOT a calorie: calories from sugar are the most harmful. Fructose, in particular, may indirectly cause high insulin levels, obesity and metabolic syndrome
- Sugar is a highly addictive substance
- Eat little or no refined sugar (watch out for hidden sugar in processed supermarket items)
- Increase the amount of fibre in your diet.

2) In a nutshell:

- A healthy diet is *not* about counting calories: it's about wholesome food choices
- It's about eating when you're hungry, and stopping when you're full
- Trust your body: it will let you know *when* and *how much* you should eat
- Your body is an amazing machine: don't underestimate it!

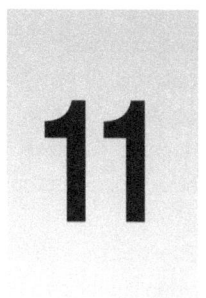

11

. . . .

TO EXERCISE OR NOT TO EXERCISE? THAT IS THE QUESTION!

. . . .

You don't need to exercise to lose weight!

Donna, a career advisor aged 53, is a size 16: ten kilograms over her healthy BMI. She's been trying to lose weight for a long time. Donna has two adult children, both studying and living at home. Her husband is a 'fly in fly out' mining engineer. Donna goes to the gym three times a week. She jogs on the treadmill for 45 minutes, and spends half an hour lifting weights. Donna eats the same, fairly balanced meals as the rest of the household. She's the only one in the family who goes to the gym, yet she's the only one who is overweight, She finds it very frustrating. Her husband and children wonder why she hasn't lost more weight, despite her dedication to exercise.

Most weight loss methods rely on a restrictive diet combined with physical exercise, but recent scientific research reveals that exercise has been overrated. Exercise has many health benefits, but the direct impact of exercise on weight loss is minimal, contrary to popular belief. Exercise with the sole intention of burning calories is an eating disorder, as it should be done for other reasons than just wanting to lose weight!

The combination of strict dieting and intense physical exertion has been the gospel of weight loss since the mid-1960s. Even though this concept is relatively recent in history, and characteristic of the 'baby-boomer' generation, it is hard to challenge, as it is deeply ingrained in our collective subconscious.

French-American scientist Jean Mayer (1920 - 1993) was best known for his research on the physiology of hunger and metabolism of essential nutrients. In the 1950s, Jean Mayer was the first researcher to introduce a link between exercise and weight reduction. Until then, the idea that physical activity may help you shed weight was actually quite unfashionable in the scientific community. In the 1930s, bed rest was even advocated as an effective way to treat obese patients!

Jen Mayer revolutionized this approach by proving that the less active someone is, the more likely they are to be overweight. As a result of his research, 'getting fit' became synonymous with healthy living and a lean body in the 60s and 70s. This paved the way for a burgeoning gym industry. As people became more and more sedentary, obesity steadily increased and it was easy to conclude that inactivity causes weight gain. But have we confused cause and effect? These days, scientists suspect that it is fatness that causes inactivity, and not the other way around. Inactivity alone does not lead to being overweight or obese.

According to the latest scientific findings, exercise only works minimally for weight loss. The rationale behind losing weight is to burn *more* calories than you ingest. This works well in theory, but not so well in practice. Two hours of vigorous cycling burns only 500 calories, which is the equivalent of two doughnuts. To lose half a kilogram, you would need to run roughly 120 kilometres, which is the driving distance from Sydney to Burradoo. You could achieve the same result by skipping dinner for just a week! Unless you have the willpower, stamina and training schedule of an Olympic athlete, exercise will do little in terms of shedding unwanted kilos.

Sweating and straining and gritting your teeth won't guarantee success. Recent scientific findings show that an intense workout at the gym is actually less effective than a moderate walk with your dog. 'Formal' exercise can be strenuous, boring, painful and repetitive. Some people feel anxious and intimidated when they have to exercise in a gym facility. It can also be time-consuming and difficult to fit into a daily routine, especially if you work full-time and have other responsibilities, or if you don't have easy access to a gym facility. It is costly, and, if you don't use your membership, you feel guilty and frustrated. You feel stressed about the wasted money, and disappointed in yourself for not adhering to the program you promised to follow. Your self-esteem suffers, which makes you want to eat more.

Food choices are important, but there are no 'good' and 'bad' foods, and there is no good or bad way to exercise. Exercise shouldn't be a chore. It shouldn't require huge amounts of willpower. Just like eating healthily, moving your body can be done in a playful, pleasant way. Eating is about nourishing your body, while enjoying tasteful cuisine. It's not about dieting and losing weight. Exercise is about finding pleasure in moving your body, not just for the sake of burning calories.

When you walk your dog, you enjoy this special time with your animal, and you feel pleased that he enjoys it too. You're physically active, but instead of being a chore, it's something you enjoy.

It's easy to make it a habit, as your dog needs to be exercised regularly. If you make something a habit, it becomes *automatic* and requires almost no willpower. Once a habit is established, it becomes a natural part of you.

Exercise can be problematic, as it makes you hungry. After a vigorous workout, your body wants to replenish burned energy. You feel ravenous. You may be tempted to give in to your cravings. You may not have enough willpower to resist these powerful, post-workout urges.

Increase the amount of complex carbohydrates and fibre in your meals and add lean protein to them: you will have more energy. An intense craving for cake or ice-cream is a sign that your blood sugar has dropped *too* low. You may even binge as a result of an exhausting workout. Some people feel that they need to reward themselves with a treat after working out.

Hunger in itself is not a bad thing; how you deal with it makes all the difference. Ignoring hunger signals because you want to burn calories indicates an eating disorder. Binging is just as dysfunctional. A functional way to eat is to respond to your body's hunger signals appropriately, with nutritious meals and snacks that you can enjoy.

You may be tempted to exercise compulsively in the hope of burning more calories and accelerating your weight loss. Over-exercising can be dangerous. As well as making you prone to injuries, it can leave you sore, dehydrated, weak, fatigued, irritable and depressed. Don't abuse yourself; love your body and respect it. Develop a moderate exercise routine that suits your ability and your needs.

A balance of exercise, rest and recreation is essential for good physical and mental health. Planned exercise should not interfere with your leisure time and social life. If you find yourself constantly obsessing about it, you may suffer from exercise addiction.

The value of rigorous exercise has been exaggerated, especially for the purpose of weight loss. A lot of people blame their lack of willpower for their inability to lose weight. The same people also believe their failure to slim down is due to a lack of exercise. 'I can't lose weight because I don't have time to exercise.' But we all have time to move a bit more, with gentle exercise like walking. Walking is the best exercise: it's cheap, effective and doesn't require special skills or equipment; just a good pair of walking shoes.

Homemakers, nurses, cleaners, waiters, sales assistants, flight attendants, trades people or labourers have physically demanding jobs. They don't need to go to the gym, as they already get plenty of exercise during their working hours. *Awareness* can change the way you think, and it can also lead to better fitness. Just being conscious that you're exercising can make a huge difference. People who recognise their work as exercise enjoy greater health benefits. Research has shown that these people experience a drop in body weight, BMI and body fat. They also have lower blood pressure and less stress than those who continue their work mindlessly, without being aware that they're exercising.

Once you become aware that your work or other activity fulfils your recommendations for daily activity levels, you feel a sense of relief. You will automatically begin to alter your lifestyle and adjust your diet, choosing more fruit and vegetables instead of fast foods full of fat, sugar and salt. A lot of people naturally enjoy moving and being active. Unless you're a complete couch potato, you don't need to over-exert yourself to burn calories. This is what your body does naturally, given the right food, and as long as your major organs, liver and kidneys, are working properly. Drinking a lot of water is also important as it helps to rid your body of toxins.

'Don't try to lose weight if you're not prepared to exercise' is what you've probably been told. But no one has ever lost weight with the help of exercise alone. Perhaps you're afraid to be a normal weight, because you think that you'll have to exercise all the time, rushing to the gym in the early hours before work or pounding the treadmill after an exhausting day.

The fear of exercise might stop you from attempting to lose weight in the first place, and you've been made to believe that it's impossible to be slim without putting a lot of effort into an exercise routine. Just like dieting, exercising can easily turn into an obsession. A diet in itself is an eating disorder, as you're only looking at the caloric content of your food. There is no enjoyment; eating becomes something you do to lose weight, and that's dysfunctional. Take your focus off dieting and exercising, as a means to restrict and exert yourself, and put it on health and wellbeing instead.

Not all normal-weight people exercise and many of them are just as 'lazy' as anyone else. Many overweight people spend several hours a week exercising, but it hasn't done much to solve their problem. Some become discouraged, as they try so hard to burn calories and fat, but it never seems to work. They lose weight just to regain it a few weeks or a few months later. They feel cheated and angry at themselves for being unable to attain an ideal shape, while simultaneously losing their confidence and self-esteem. They might decide to exercise even more vigorously or to restrict their food intake even further, the perfect setup for a binge.

Don't torture yourself. Feeling good is more important than being skinny. You have been taught to fight *against* everything, in the hope of overcoming it – but what you resist will persist. Instead, you can let go of what is preventing you from enjoying true wellbeing. What stops you from being a healthy weight is your inability to *release* what is making you fat. This journey is not about losing or winning the 'Battle of the Bulge'. It's about being in tune with your body and responding to its signals adequately. If you listen to it, your body will tell you what it needs, whether it is food or exercise.

Just like food, exercise can only make you feel good if there is no guilt attached to it; that is, if it's a free choice, not something you're *forced* to do. Just like a crash diet, a rigid exercise program is like a jail sentence, a punishment. You can't wait to escape from it. If you feel forced to exercise against your will, and even if you're the only one forcing yourself, you will rebel. Your rebellion will take the form of bingeing or giving up exercise altogether, which often means giving up *all* intention of losing weight.

If you have to put tremendous effort into what you're doing, you won't be able to keep it up for long. Rather than using willpower to force yourself to do something, it's easier to carry out actions because they come to you naturally. If you eat healthily every day without feeling hungry and deprived, you will enjoy it, as it is what you want. Healthy meals and snacks will become a set of habits, an integral part of your daily routine.

To replace compulsive eating with compulsive exercising doesn't help. Don't rely on exercise to lose weight or maintain your current weight. You won't trust your body, and you won't trust yourself. You will rely on something *external* to you, instead of relying on your *own* inner strength. You will feel guilt and discomfort if you don't submit to your daily exercise routine, and, secretly, you will resent it. To move your body should give you pleasure, not pain.

As your circumstances change, you may not be able to exercise for various reasons. You may become sick or injured. You may become too busy, due to a promotion, a new job or other commitments, or you may no longer be able to afford your gym membership.

If you exercise religiously and obsess about it, you'll feel bad as soon as you miss a session. You may want to exercise to alleviate your guilt. By punishing yourself that way, you believe that you can redeem yourself and make up for your dietary 'sins'. Eating and emotions are intimately connected. If you think you've blown it by eating the wrong food or not submitting to your daily workout, you feel as if you have failed. You might even decide to stuff yourself with food and forget about your diet until the next day!

If you expect to stick to a strict exercise routine, you're likely to fail. But without expectations, there can be no failure. Don't expect anything of yourself, and you won't be disappointed. Every day you have choices. You could choose to eat junk food all day, or you could opt for fresh, nutrient-rich, healthy, low-fat foods. Fresh fruit, vegetables and complex carbohydrates will fill you up, leaving little room for junk food. You can choose to exercise today, as you know it will make you feel better, or you can decide to relax in front of the TV instead. It won't be the end of the world. Recreation is just as important as work, and you can't make efforts all the time.

Stop feeling guilt, the 'useless emotion'. Guilt is feeling bad about something you've done in the past. Why worry about actions you've got no control over? Perhaps what you did was wrong, but placing the burden of guilt on yourself will only make it worse. Guilt is a negative emotion, and it is destructive. Don't beat yourself up about mistakes you've made. View them as learning opportunities instead. Don't have any expectations, as you will feel guilty if you fail to meet them. This could result in a cycle of bingeing or over-exercising or simply giving up.

Guilt causes stress and fear, and it sets you up for failure even before you've started. Accepting responsibility is okay, but guilt is a waste of time, and punishing yourself won't help. You're allowed *not* to exercise if you don't feel like it. And you're allowed to have fun! Listen to your *real* self, not the bossy voice in your head that tells you to get up and go to the gym, no matter how you feel.

A lot of activities are not strenuous, but you still benefit from the gentle workout they provide. You don't have to be sweating, out of breath and your heart pounding in order to be fit. Walking, housework, gardening, window-shopping or washing your car are physical tasks that are good for you, and they contribute towards your daily exercise quota.

If you have children or grandchildren, you have a never-ending supply of activities that will keep you fit and agile. A park, a public swimming pool or a suburban backyard can provide opportunities to improve your fitness while having a laugh and bonding with your kids. Observe children and notice how they love to play, how they take pleasure in moving their bodies. By joining in their fun, you can learn from them, and happy times shared together will be fond memories.

Every day, you can look for opportunities to move a bit more. You can use the stairs; you can walk or cycle to work. You can stroll to the corner store instead of taking the car. Use public transport; it will save you money and it will help protect the environment by reducing greenhouse gases and traffic jams. And you'll get some exercise, as you'll have to walk to the bus or train station and back.

Don't reject exercise altogether because of your apprehension or your negative experiences. There can't be any failure if there are no expectations. You don't have to be a slave to your routine. Between ten and thirty minutes of moderate exercise daily could be enough to improve your wellbeing. The best time to exercise is in the morning, as it will boost your metabolism and lift your spirits.

Exercise is a natural anti-depressant. It stimulates the production of serotonin and endorphins, and you will feel calm and focused. Be playful and make it fun. Find something you enjoy but don't overdo it, as too much exercise can be harmful: it affects your metabolism and immune system in a negative way. As with all things, moderation is the key.

Positive aspects of moderate exercise:

Exercise may not be as effective as we thought to control weight, but it has many other health benefits. A lot of conditions could be prevented or improved with regular activity:

- Exercise increases your metabolic rate: you burn more energy, and the effect lasts up to several hours after the workout has stopped
- It helps you gain muscle and reshape your body, giving it a firmer, more 'toned' aspect
- It's a good way to 'detox' as it stimulates your liver and kidneys, especially if you drink plenty of water
- It's a good way to socialize and make friends with like-minded people
- Exercise boosts your *self-esteem*, as you gain a sense of control and confidence
- Exercise prevents high blood pressure, high cholesterol, heart disease, type 2 diabetes, osteoporosis, osteoarthritis and even cancer
- For people with diabetes, physical activity improves the body's response to *insulin*, which lowers blood sugar levels
- Exercise stimulates the digestive tract and relieves *constipation,* especially when combined with a high fibre diet
- Exercise increases your resistance to infections, as it boosts the immune system

- Regular, *low* impact exercise is a natural *anti-depressant*
- Exercise reduces stress, gives you more energy, and improves the quality of your sleep.
- It helps relieve back, shoulder and neck pain (especially if you swim, do yoga or tai chi)
- For older people: regular exercise prevents Alzheimer's disease, as it improves blood circulation to the *brain*. It makes you stronger, more agile and better able to move around without falling. It also makes it easier for you to perform daily activities such as gardening or vacuuming

Key Points and Strategies:

- Be in tune with your body and listen to its signals
- Over-exercising can be detrimental to your health
- Exercise will make you hungry, so fill up on nutritious food to avoid cravings
- Don't feel guilty if you miss out on a workout session
- If you're physically active at work, be *aware* of it, as it may be enough to fulfil your daily exercise requirements
- Design a flexible, gentle exercise routine that suits your needs
- Do some housework or gardening if you don't like going to gym
- Walk more often, and increase distance and pace as you get fitter if you wish to
- Ten to thirty minutes a day of low impact exercise is all you need
- Have fun exercising and enjoy moving your body.

12

. . . .

BOOST YOUR METABOLISM

. . . .

Activate your metabolism and burn fat effectively.

Carmen, 43, has been dieting since her early thirties. Every six to eight months, she goes on a strict diet combined with vigorous exercise. She loses between ten and fifteen kilograms. She then quits her diet and regains all her weight within the next few months.

Like so many yo-yo dieters, Carmen has three sets of clothes: 'fat', 'skinny' and a few different sizes in between. Her big clothes are baggy and tasteless; her skinny wardrobe is elegant and fashionable. Carmen lives for the magic moment when she will be slim once and for all, and wear her small-sized garments all the time.

She finds it more and more difficult to lose weight and to keep it off. No matter how hard she tries, the figure on the scale won't budge. She now weighs 82 kilograms, and it's the heaviest she's ever been. She eats almost nothing during the day, but has a big evening meal. She avoids carbohydrates most of the time, as she thinks they're too fattening.

Carmen has lost all hope of losing weight. She believes that her metabolism is too slow and that her body won't cooperate. She believes that her body stubbornly wants to remain fat, despite her best intentions. She would still like to lose weight, but she doesn't think she can do it without a magic wand. Carmen feels like a failure and doesn't want to get out of bed in the morning any more. Lately she finds herself eating chocolate and ice cream more often.

Yo-yo dieting, also called 'weight cycling' is the repeated loss and regain of body weight. According to scientific studies and contrary to popular belief, yo-yo dieting does *not* slow your metabolism. It doesn't make it harder to lose weight in the future. But it can be harmful to your health, as it has been linked to certain risks such as high cholesterol and high blood pressure. Losing and regaining weight has a negative psychological effect, as you may become discouraged and depressed and turn to food for emotional reasons.

Fad diets don't work due to their *rebound* effect. To lose weight permanently, you need to commit yourself to lifelong changes in your eating and activity pattern. These changes are not difficult to implement if you understand the reasoning behind them. Blaming your inability to lose weight on a sluggish metabolism doesn't help. A few techniques will help you overcome this problem and kick start your weight loss. If you're a man you have an advantage, as men naturally have a faster metabolism than women: it's easier for them to shed body fat. *Age* is also a big factor and, once you're over 40, your metabolism is a lot slower than when you were half that age.

According to science, there are only two proven ways to speed up your metabolism: increasing the body's muscle mass and increasing the body's heart rate. Blood is pushed through your body with every heartbeat, and the best way to raise your heart rate is to *exercise.* Although exercise on its own may only have a minimal effect on weight loss, it is a good way to rev up your metabolism. Together with a healthy diet, it can create the synergy needed for successful weight loss.

Metabolism includes all the processes that occur within the body and that are designed to keep you alive. Your basal metabolism is the energy you require to function while at rest. You use up more energy when you're active. Weight loss can be difficult because you need to spend *more* energy than you take in from food. While your aim is to lose fat, you want to preserve and develop your muscles. When there is insufficient muscle tissue, you burn less energy, which is a good reason to exercise moderately and tone your body.

Your metabolism dictates the rate at which energy is burnt in your body, and how fast your fat stores diminish when you're dieting. Some people enjoy a fast metabolism, and seem to be able to eat anything without getting fat. Some underweight people have trouble putting on weight. They have to force themselves to eat, just to maintain their current shape, or they would be too skinny. Such people are more the exception than the rule. Most of us have the opposite problem: we seem to burn calories too slowly and store fat too easily. Sometimes our metabolism is so energy-efficient (something desirable in a home or a kitchen appliance) that we don't seem to lose any weight at all, even though we drastically reduce our food intake. Some of us are so good at conserving energy that we would do well during a famine!

When your metabolism is too slow, your body refuses to burn fat, no matter how much effort you put into losing weight. As time goes by, the problem seems to worsen instead of resolving itself. As you mature, you need to eat less – just when you're developing an interest in cooking, tasting food and gastronomy! Your need for dietary fat also diminishes with age. Children require a higher percentage of fat in their diet. As they're growing, they need more concentrated supplies of energy in the form of fatty acids. Fat is also important for the developing nervous system (brain and nerves). This is especially true for babies and toddlers, and breast milk is surprisingly high in fat.

Pregnancy increases your metabolic rate as the body needs to cater for the needs of the growing foetus. This is not a good time to lose weight, and it generally doesn't happen anyway, as most women will experience an increase in appetite and cravings, due to pregnancy hormones – sometimes even insatiable hunger. This is how the body ensures that enough nutrients reach the foetus.

What causes your metabolism to slow down?

- Skipping meals: your body thinks that it might have to prepare for famine, causing it to lower its metabolism in an effort to save energy (starvation mode)
- Fasting: while eating increases your metabolism, fasting decreases it
- Not enough calories: your body goes into starvation mode
- Too much or not enough exercise
- Too much or not enough sleep
- Not drinking enough water
- Menopause (change of life)
- Chronic stress.

Initially, *stress* may increase your metabolic rate, as it causes your heart to beat faster. But eventually, it will make you fat, due to an excessive production of the stress hormone *cortisone,* along with a reduced secretion of several other key hormones. Chronic, persistent stress causes the body to store fat and lose muscle, while the metabolism decreases and appetite increases. Overall, stress makes you burn fewer calories and consume more food (especially sweet items), which increases your stress levels even more.

What is stress?

Stress is fear, anxiety: the ominous feeling of not being able to cope with what life dishes out to you. Take a few deep breaths and *relax*. Think about how you could improve your daily routine. Plan ahead and design a 'To Do List'. Write it down in your diary. *Prioritise* if you feel overwhelmed. Certain tasks are more important than others. Eating nutritious meals should be your number one priority, as well as incorporating some gentle exercise in your weekly schedule.

Know your limits and don't take on too much. Learn how to say no, and don't be a people-pleaser. Delegate as much as possible to others and trust that they can do it. You might be the best at cleaning the house, but, if you don't ask your children to do it, they will never have the opportunity to give it a go. They might not do a very good job, but does it really matter? The more they do it, the better they will be at it.

Empty your mind and let things go. Nothing will ever be exactly how you would like it to be. If you reconcile yourself with your circumstances, and live in the present with an attitude of gratefulness, you'll pave the way for good things to come. Don't obsess about results; enjoy *processes* and let go of outcomes. Spend more quality time with your family and your pets. See the funny side of things. Lightening up will lighten your burden!

Cravings are associated with certain brain chemicals. As humans, we have evolved to associate high calorie foods with pleasure and enjoyment. On the negative side, *stress* promotes cravings, as it means that energy has been burned up. This was true in the past, when humans had to physically face danger or run away from it. These days, stress is a mental thing, but the body responds in the same way. We crave sugar and fat to replace lost calories as quickly as possible and feel 'normal' again.

A medical check-up is a good way to eliminate physical causes when all your weight loss efforts seem to be in vain. Excessive dieting has a harmful effect on your metabolism. Your body is programmed to conserve fat, not to eliminate it, so it will ring the alarm bells as soon as your caloric intake becomes too low. The less you eat, the less energy you'll burn, especially if you drastically reduce your carbohydrate intake.

Due to strong peer pressure and the ideal of a model-like figure promoted by the media, teenage girls often diet, even though they're already slim. A lot of young people believe that in order to be attractive, they need to be as thin as a super model, famous actor or sports person. Unfortunately, celebrities often suffer from eating disorders, which is not something youngsters should emulate. Dieting when not overweight is harmful, as it has a negative effect on your metabolism, slowing it down.

A sluggish metabolism may be difficult to reverse once it has set in as a result of repeated crash diets. You risk ending up overweight, even though your weight was normal to begin with. One of the most famous and harmful comments uttered by a celebrity was, 'You can never be too rich or too thin' (Wallis Simpson, Duchess of Windsor) This is. the equivalent of promoting eating disorders. It is a careless attitude towards a problem that many people have to deal with for years and sometimes for a lifetime. Of course, you *can* be too thin, and it's just as harmful as being overweight or obese. Dieting can definitely make you fat. This is especially true if you don't need to diet in the first place, or if you cut calories and carbs too low and do too much exercise.

Moderate exercise will gently stimulate a sluggish metabolism, but over-exercising has the opposite effect. If you exercise too much, your body will only burn a minimum of calories, in order to preserve energy. There is a rebound effect after discontinuing vigorous exercise. Your metabolism will automatically slow down if you revert to your couch potato lifestyle, after you've exerted yourself for several hours a day on a regular basis. The combination of strenuous exercise and drastic, low-carb dieting has the most detrimental effect on your fat-burning mechanism. It effectively conditions the body to hang on to its fat stores!

A lack of complex carbohydrates will make you feel hungry, which sets you up for strong cravings. It also depletes your brain of *serotonin,* leaving you anxious, nervous and irritable. Carbohydrates are the body's natural fuel. Fat and protein also provide energy, but with carbs, this energy is more readily available. Carbohydrates help increase your metabolism, as they stimulate the active processes in your body and promote fat-burning. Eating only steak and lettuce doesn't work: you need to add *slow* carbs to your diet, such as brown rice, wholemeal pasta, beans or potatoes. These 'good' carbs will stop you from feeling hungry and stressed.

To prevent hunger attacks and help your body burn fat, have several small meals, rather than three big ones. Small meals ensure you have a constant supply of energy for your physical and mental needs. To spread your calories throughout the day is a balanced way to eat, and it has been proven to speed up weight loss.

Your metabolism varies, depending on what time of the day it is. A lot of diets don't take into consideration that you burn more calories in the morning than in the evening. Using this principle to your advantage, you can eat more and lose weight at the same time! *When* you eat is just as crucial as *what* you eat it. You would lose weight more easily if you ate your meals earlier.

Are you a night-time eater? Maybe you eat most of your calories late in the evening, when the 'fat-burning factory' is not operational. Maybe you have a habit of skipping breakfast, missing out on a time of the day when most calories are burnt instead of being stored as fat. When you eat too late and have big meals at night, you're not in harmony with your body clock and you'll sabotage your own weight loss efforts. This type of eating pattern creates an imbalance; your metabolism slows down as a result.

Your biological clock has a big impact on your health and how your body burns calories and fat. Different hormones are released into your bloodstream at different hours of the day and night, affecting your mood, your wellbeing and your metabolism. If you're not in tune with your biological clock, your metabolism will be sluggish or even stagnant.

A chocolate bar at 10 a.m. is not the same as a chocolate bar at 10 p.m. Your body is designed to burn energy in the morning. At night, the system shuts down to prepare you for sleep. Everything slows down and calorie-burning almost comes to a halt, which is why all the calories you eat at night are stored as fat, especially those coming from saturated fats, trans-fats and sugar. In the morning, the process is reversed: your body is programmed to burn energy, and almost everything you eat before midday will be used as fuel.

Take advantage of your body's natural tendency to burn energy in the morning. If you starve all day, a big splurge is almost inevitable in the evening, and your craving for high-calorie foods will be irresistible. Some people eat non-stop from the time they get home from work until they collapse in bed!

Do you complain that you can't lose weight, even though you don't eat much? It may be true, if you consider calories alone. But if you have a habit of eating late in the day, your metabolism slows down. No matter what you do, you won't be able to shift your weight. Out of all the meals you consume, dinner is the most fattening, especially if it is a late dinner with a lot of animal protein, fat and sugar. If possible, eat dinner *early* in the evening and make it *light* and palatable. For instance, you could have:

- Low-fat cottage cheese, raw vegetables (e.g. tomato, capsicum, cucumber, spring onion) and wholemeal bread
- Steamed vegetables and prawns with brown rice
- Corn, avocado and chick pea salad with crusty wholemeal bread
- Homemade tomato soup with wholemeal noodles
- Grilled low-fat cheese on rye bread with spring onion, lettuce, tomato and beetroot
- Broiled fish, baked potato, peas and carrots
- Fresh fruit salad, plain Greek yoghurt and low-fat crackers
- Stir fried vegetables with chicken breast and brown rice
- Roast turkey breast, green beans and broiled tomatoes
- Lean beef strips, broccoli and sweet potato
- Chicken Teriyaki with vegetables and wholemeal noodles
- Shaved Brussels sprouts salad with fresh nuts and low-fat grated cheese
- Tofu burger and tossed salad with balsamic vinegar
- Wholemeal pasta and lentil sauce with onion, garlic and tomato, topped with reduced-fat feta
- Pumpkin soup and veggie burrito

- Apple and onion baked chicken with steamed spinach and a few cashews
- Minestrone with a little grated Parmesan cheese.

Skip the glass of wine or evening cocktail with dinner. Only drink water or herbal tea without sugar or milk. Go to your local library and browse the healthy recipe book section, or Google the internet for delicious light recipes and endless mouth-watering combinations: you'll find countless recipe websites at the click of a mouse, and most of them offer low-calorie, as well as vegetarian, options.

Key Points and Strategies:

- Increase your body's muscle mass and your heart rate with moderate exercise
- Avoid strict dieting and excessive vigorous exercise, as it will slow your metabolism
- Avoid weight cycling and 'yo-yo' dieting, but don't let past failures discourage you
- Avoid stress by planning ahead and prioritising, while letting go of outcomes
- Don't go on a diet if your BMI is within the normal range
- Have carbohydrate-rich meals to prevent hunger pangs and activate your metabolism
- Spread your calories throughout the days by having several small meals
- Take time to plan and prepare a light, nutritious and tasty dinner
- Google healthy recipe for inspiration and ideas
- If possible, eat all your calories before the sun goes down.

13

THE IMPORTANCE OF EATING BREAKFAST

Eat a wholesome breakfast: it's the best way to fuel your day while losing weight

Your internal biological clock regulates your metabolism. You tend to burn energy at a speedy rate in the morning and during the active part of your day. After that, your metabolism progressively slows down, almost coming to a standstill in the late evening, before you get ready for sleep. Your metabolism is slowest at night when you sleep, and in the morning before you eat.

This pattern is based on your activity levels generally being higher during the day. People who work odd hours – nurses, ambulance or police officers, those who do the 'graveyard shift' – constantly struggle as they go *against* their body's natural rhythm. Most organisms have evolved to coordinate their activities with the day and night cycle caused by the earth's rotation. Biological clocks have evolved to time biological processes. Your circadian clock regulates many aspects of your behaviour and physiology, including your metabolism. It will decide whether it's time to burn energy or to store it for later use.

To keep your metabolism raised, you need to eat *small* meals, if possible every three to four hours throughout the day, rather than three large ones. The best way to keep your metabolism elevated is to keep the fuel going, and to ensure you eat several high-quality small meals a day.

Breakfast plays a major role in starting up your metabolism. If you don't bother with the most important meal of your day, your metabolism will remain slow for the rest of the day. At night, fuel consumption is at its lowest and the only way to start it up again is to eat breakfast.

'Eat breakfast like a king, lunch like a prince and dinner like a pauper' – this common saying is not outdated: it's supported by recent scientific research. Two groups of a few hundred people each were given exactly the same amount of calories during the day. People in the first group had their biggest meal at lunchtime, while people in the other group had theirs in the evening. The group that ate most of their calories early in the day lost considerably more weight than those who ate their biggest meal late in the evening.

Begin your day with a full, balanced and healthy meal. As the hours tick by, eat *lighter* meals and *smaller* portions, especially as you're moving towards the evening. You will sleep well, without feeling too full, and without feeling hungry, especially if you've stocked up on slow carbohydrates earlier in the day. Your metabolism will continue to work efficiently while you sleep and be ready the next morning for another cycle.

Do you often feel you're running on empty most of the time? Does your energy level drop when you reach the middle of the day? Do you experience a mid-afternoon slump, when all you want to do is rest your head on the desk, wondering how you'll survive the rest of the day? Your brain and muscles need *glucose* to function, and, if you've skipped breakfast, you're off to a bad start. You're almost sure to 'crash', possibly even before lunchtime.

Studies have shown that children and teenagers who eat breakfast have a better attitude than those who don't. They get less tired and cranky during the day. They perform better during tests or exams, understand and absorb new concepts more easily and have a longer attention span. The same is true for adults. Eating breakfast will enable you to be more enthusiastic and more active during the day. It increases your energy levels. It will boost your metabolism, and you'll be more inclined to be physically active.

You'll be more likely to go for a walk after work if you don't feel exhausted. Breakfast is the cornerstone of your diet, and it will set the mood for the entire day. The foods you eat play an important role for weight loss and for your wellbeing. The right kind of food can keep you satiated and vitalised for the whole morning and possibly for the rest of the day. It will make you less likely to splurge on sugary treats later on.

The ideal breakfast is a combination of protein and complex carbohydrates with fibre. Include protein like whole eggs, lean ham, tofu, baked beans, yoghourt or ricotta cheese with a sprinkle of *nuts* and *seeds*. Have fresh *fruit* (berries and bananas go well with yoghourt and porridge) and whole grain breads or cereal, preferably *oats,* as they have a very low GI (Corn flakes have a very high GI and it's best to restrict them). Eating *whole grains*, especially first thing in the morning, will keep your blood sugar constant, and will give you more energy throughout the day.

Drink at least eight glasses of water a day, as this will boost your metabolism and energy levels. Your aim is not only to lose weight, but to maintain your drive and your productivity as a human being. You want to be fit for your daily activities. If you feel sluggish and irritable, you won't be motivated to maintain your weight loss efforts. Ultimately, the success of your diet will depend on the quality of your breakfast.

Some people say they haven't had breakfast for years and it hasn't affected them negatively. Of course, no one will starve or have serious health issues if they skip breakfast. But, if you have your last meal around 7 p.m. and get up early in the morning, your body has to go a long time without food. By then you will be ready for a decent meal to 'break the fast', which will keep your energy and blood glucose levels optimal.

Lunch is equally important. Along with *vegetables* (raw or cooked) and *protein* like tuna, tofu, lean poultry, ham or nut butter, your lunch should include a portion of complex carbs with high fibre content: wholegrain or rye bread, plain oatcakes, bean or lentil soup, brown rice or wholemeal pasta in a salad or with steamed vegetables.

Imagine a fire: when you first light it, it burns fast and high. Everything you add to it will be consumed quickly by its flames. First thing in the morning, your body is a calorie-burning machine. If you skip breakfast, you will miss out on the *least* fattening meal of the day. Eating breakfast will instantly add fuel to your fire and accelerate your metabolism. If you don't eat breakfast, your metabolism will remain *slow* and continue to slow down as the day progresses. Give yourself a good start by planning ahead for a nutritious breakfast.

Go to bed at a reasonable time to avoid fatigue, and have everything you need ready for the morning. Set your alarm twenty minutes before your usual wake up time and don't press the snooze button. Rising early gives you extra time to get ready without rushing. Don't get side-tracked; focus on what you're doing and keep in time. If you have trouble getting up, put your alarm out of reach, somewhere across the room, so you need to get up to turn it off. Looking forward to your breakfast will motivate you to get up and stay up. Leave your bedroom and have a glass of water. Stretch or do some physical exercise for a few minutes: this will help you get moving. Have a shower, get dressed and... enjoy a healthy breakfast!

The night before, as part of your bedtime routine, set up your breakfast dishes, hot water kettle or coffee machine, and make sure you have all the ingredients on hand: low fat milk or soy milk, oats, nuts, seeds, rye bread, fresh fruit, berries, eggs, tomatoes, cottage cheese, lean ham or vegetarian substitute.

Good planning is half your work done, and it is your staircase to success. 'By failing to prepare, you are preparing to fail', said Benjamin Franklin, and this applies to most life situations. Breakfast only takes a few minutes to plan, by including certain items on your shopping list and storing them in your fridge and kitchen cupboard. It only takes a few minutes to prepare your meal and clean up after yourself.

Leave for work or other activity five to ten minutes earlier than you need to. Stick to your new morning routine for at least 21 days. On weekends, don't sleep in or stay up too late, to avoid disturbing your body clock and metabolism. At least don't sleep more than one or two hours past your usual wake up time, and keep to your average bedtime as much as possible.

It only takes 21 days to form a new habit. This has been evidenced by research: your brain requires this amount of time to develop new pathways. Once the neural connections are in place, they will function automatically. Now you're on auto-pilot, as the new habit has become a natural part of you. You won't need as much willpower and self-discipline as in the beginning to adhere to your new routine. After three weeks, you will notice the benefits from your new habit, which will be an incentive for your subconscious mind to continue that way.

Instead of saying to yourself, 'I have to do this for the rest of my life', decide to do it for 21 days only, and see what happens afterwards. If even a 21 day period appears too daunting, try the one-day-at-a-time approach. This is an ancient philosophy that has become popular with Twelve Step groups. Living a day at a time doesn't mean you will be disorganised and leave things to chance. You can live for this day only, while planning for the next.

What if you never have breakfast because you don't feel hungry in the morning? The reason you're not hungry is that you never eat at that time, so you've conditioned your body not to expect any nourishment. As a result, your body has adapted and doesn't send out hunger signals. Your body has learnt to keep its metabolism down to a minimum until it is given food. It remains slow until you eat, which generally happens mid-morning, when you ravenously devour your morning tea muffins, or at lunchtime. In the worst case scenario you won't feel hungry until the evening and have a big dinner followed by unhealthy snacks in front of the TV.

If you reverse this pattern and start eating in the morning, your body will soon respond accordingly. Your metabolism *will* accelerate, and you will begin to feel hungry as soon as you get out of bed. Hunger is the reflection of a healthy metabolism: it means you're burning calories. Eating uses up energy, as food is digested before it is metabolised. This is why eating frequently is effective in raising your metabolism.

Some people may never feel hungry in the morning no matter what they do to condition themselves, but just because you're not starving doesn't mean you shouldn't eat anything. Even if you were lying in bed all day, you would still use up calories to keep your organs functioning. After a night's rest, your stomach is empty, but it may not be sending out signals because it hasn't quite woken up yet. Even though you don't feel the need for it, your body requires nourishment. If you don't eat breakfast, you'll soon be running on empty. Your car won't start on an empty tank, but you expect your body to do it.

Introducing a new habit can be tricky, as we tend to resist changes, at least in the beginning. I advise to do it *progressively*. If you're not a 'breakfast person', you won't be able to change overnight. Start by introducing small amounts of food: a piece of wholemeal toast with a slice of melted cheese or an apple, or a small serve of porridge topped with a few berries. Steadily increase the amount of food you eat for breakfast over the next three weeks. Eat slightly less at lunch and dinner, while having regular healthy snacks in between meals.

Record how you feel in your diary. You'll soon find that you're less hungry during the day and have more energy. You'll be more efficient at your work or studies. You'll be able to cope better with pressure and mental stress. You'll be able to think more clearly and positively. You'll be more pleasant and patient with people around you. You'll be more grateful for all the little things you used to take for granted, and you'll notice them more often.

When running on empty, you're not aware of your surroundings, or you only pay attention to what you *don't* like; you find fault with everything and everyone. You play the blame game: it's someone else's fault, or it's the situation you're in. Without breakfast, your morning gets off to a bad start and will only get worse. But once you've eaten breakfast consistently for 21 days, you'll experience a positive change. The world will be a friendlier place, right from the time you get up. As the day progresses, you'll be more likely to remain in a positive frame of mind. And you won't feel drained by the time you get home. You'll still have enough energy to put on your sneakers and go for a run or a walk.

Refrain from drinking too much coffee, as it lowers your blood sugar. If you need two or three coffees to wake up, you probably didn't get enough *quality* sleep. Reassess your sleep hygiene and take steps to ensure yourself a good night's sleep. Cut down on alcohol or eliminate it altogether, as it can severely disrupt your sleep pattern. The same applies to nicotine and other drugs. A rested body and mind helps you resist temptation and stick to a sensible diet. A good night's sleep stimulates your metabolism and enhances your wellbeing and outlook on life.

Skipping breakfast is harmful, but avoiding dinner is not necessarily a bad thing, as long as you're not hungry, and as long as you've had a good breakfast and lunch, as well as some nutritious snacks. While it's okay to enjoy the occasional chocolate bar, piece of cake or cookie, make a decision not to have them late in the evening or at night. As your body relaxes and prepares for sleep, it is not geared towards burning energy any more. A *light* dinner is advisable. When eating out, prepare yourself mentally by rehearsing your choices. Stick to salads, vegetables and crudités as much as possible and drink sparkling water instead of wine or beer.

You may be reluctant to reverse your eating pattern, for fear of being out of control and putting on weight, and for fear of not being able to sleep on an empty stomach. Be reassured. Your body uses a lot of energy in the morning, and a large breakfast won't make you gain weight. On the contrary: it will rev up your metabolism. You'll enjoy better self-control as your blood sugar levels won't drop but will remain constant, so you won't experience sudden cravings. If you eat enough healthy food during the day, a small dinner will be enough to satisfy your hunger. You'll sleep better after a light evening meal, and wake up more refreshed in the morning.

Eat only when you're hungry, and you will soon realize that it's better to leave the table satisfied, but not necessarily full. To leave the table with room for more food may be difficult, especially in the evening. You look at this evening meal as your reward for a hard day's work. You've conditioned yourself to go to sleep on an overfull stomach, even if it means taking an antacid tablet at bedtime. But having room for *more* doesn't equate being hungry; it's just your appetite telling you to keep eating.

Appetite is a desire, not a need, and you can choose to give in to it or not. Be mindful while you're eating: *listen* to your body and STOP as soon as you've had enough. Put your knife and fork down between each bite to slow yourself down. Eating slowly and consciously means eating less. This awareness will prevent you from losing control. In the end, it only takes a split second to make the decision to cease eating, and place your fork and knife across your plate!

Ask yourself if all your physical and emotional needs have been met. You might be using food as a substitute, when you feel an uncontrollable urge to continue eating during or after your evening meal. Find other ways to *nurture* yourself. Relax and take time for yourself: do something you enjoy. Relaxation is not a frivolous pleasure: it is vital for your wellbeing. Sometimes you're so busy making other people happy that you forget what makes *you* happy. If you don't know how to relax, think about what you used to do when you were younger and had more free time. It's a great way to recharge your batteries.

You may be passionate about your work, or measure your self-worth by how much you accomplish in the day, but you also need to unwind. Life is a *balance* and there is a time for everything. Saying you don't need to relax is like saying you don't need to eat or sleep. Relaxation is just as important as work or exercise, and you can do it *without* technology. Instead of turning on the TV or the computer, turn them *off*. Take some deep breaths, meditate, read a page of an inspirational book. Do some baking, gardening, painting, woodwork, sewing or knitting. Do some scales if you play a musical instrument. Repetitive activities have a hypnotic effect. Above all, don't remind yourself of how much you still need to do. Let go of worries and anxiety: your brain needs a break too!

Maybe you're scared of using up all your calories before the evening. To you, eating is like budgeting, so you skip breakfast and feel in control, believing you've done the right thing. Then you wonder why you can't lose weight, blind to the fact that you're sabotaging your own weight loss efforts. When you don't eat breakfast, your metabolism slows down even before it has a chance to take off. Your body strives to *conserve* energy instead of burning it. You feel miserable all day, and ask yourself why you want to eat so much in the evening! All the calories put aside during the day might not be enough to satisfy your excruciating hunger pains.

A more sensible way to lose weight is to have a big breakfast, moderate lunch, a light dinner and small nutritious snacks in between. Foods rich in complex carbohydrates eaten during the day will still give you energy in the evening, enough to sustain you and to make a big dinner unnecessary. You *will* be able to go to sleep, and you will wake up refreshed and looking forward to your first and most important meal of the day: BREAKFAST.

Key Points and Strategies:

- Breakfast is the most important meal of the day
- Eat a substantial breakfast made of protein, complex carbohydrates and fibre
- Include fresh fruit in your first meal of the day▪ If you're not used to eating breakfast, condition yourself to do it: start small and add food slowly but gradually
- Eat a nutritious lunch and a light evening meal
- Have small healthy snacks during the day to give you energy and keep your metabolism raised ▪ Avoid eating late at night
- Don't save all your calories for the evening
- Be *focused* when you eat dinner and learn when to stop
- Don't snack mindlessly in front of the TV
- Learn how to relax *without* technology
- Eating breakfast will make you sharp, alert, calm and energetic
- It will help you lose weight and it will change your life as you'll adopt a positive outlook.

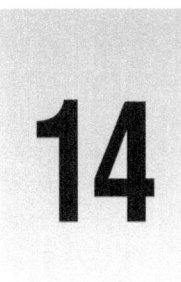

14

FAT IS GOOD FOR YOU!

Eating fat as part of a healthy diet will help you lose weight.

In the 1970s Dr Atkins published his 'Diet Revolution'. The idea that carbs were bad for you became popular and it is still fashionable today. The theory behind low-carb, high-protein and high-fat diets is to switch the body's metabolism from using glucose as energy to converting stored body fat to energy, thus promoting weight loss without having to restrict your caloric intake. You can eat as much fat and protein as you like, but *no* or very few carbs. This type of diet has many names and variations, like the Dukan diet which advocates cutting down fat as well as carbs, while solely relying on animal protein and a few greens.

Eating as much fat and protein as you wish and losing weight simultaneously sounds good, but it can be harmful. It can exacerbate your blood triglycerides and cholesterol, as well as putting extra strain on your liver and kidneys. It can increase your risk for colon cancer as it lacks fibre. Animal protein is totally devoid of fibre, as opposed to plant protein found in legumes and whole grain cereals.

Ketosis is the fat-burning state your body goes into while on this restrictive regime. It can cause *metabolic acidosis*, a dysfunctional body state characterized by blood acidity. It is usually a sign of an underlying disease, and the symptoms are: rapid breathing, nausea, confusion and lethargy. You have *no* energy and your brain is muddled up. You feel yuck. Another problem with low carb diets is that your body may start breaking down your own muscles for energy in the absence of proper fuel.

You can effectively lose weight on a low-carb diet, but ultimately it won't be good for you, as your health and vitality decline. For a diet to work, you need to be able to keep it up for the rest of your life. This is impossible with a low-carb diet, as it makes you feel dreadful. In human trials, it has been shown to inhibit mental and physical performance.

In 1979, Nathan Pritikin's diet book was published and sparked another revolution. Many Atkins 'refugees' were convinced his method held the *true* answer to permanent weight loss and wellbeing. Put off by the unpleasant side effects of the Atkins diet, they were looking for a better alternative.

Pritikin had experienced his own health challenge: he had previously been diagnosed with heart disease, which motivated him to go on a low-fat, high-fibre diet and begin a moderate exercise program. He was able to cure his condition and as a result he wrote *The Pritikin Program for Diet and Exercise*.

At first glance, Pritikin's principles make sense as he promotes unprocessed, fibre-rich foods like fresh fruit, vegetables, beans and whole grains. Pritikin pioneered the idea that there is a connection between diet and cholesterol, at a time when many doctors still believed there was no relationship. Pritikin's diet looks more reasonable than Atkins', but it is only the lesser of two evils, as it is too restrictive, cutting fat and calories way too low.

On the other hand, high protein diets like the Atkins diet encourage nutrient dense foods. On the downside, however, they may increase the risk of chronic diseases and health problems such as kidney stones, heart and gastrointestinal problems. High protein diets also lead to osteoporosis and fractures, by creating an acid environment that causes calcium to leach from your bones.

As opposed to Atkins, Pritikin recommended a low-calorie, ultra low-fat diet, which can also be the road to disaster. His diet is almost completely vegetarian and encourages the consumption of large amounts of whole grains and vegetables. It is high in fibre, which is an advantage, and low in cholesterol. It only contains 5 -7 % of total daily calories as fat, when you need to eat at least 20-35 % of your calories as fat to be healthy!

Pritikin's diet is grossly deficient in fat, but his ideas had a big impact in the 1980s and 1990s. Everything had to be fat free and you didn't dare have anything but skim milk in your coffee. Egg yolks were scorned, and you had to be out of your mind to even think about using butter! In the 2000s, things began to shift. Scientists demonstrated that not all fats had the same effect on the body: trans-fats increase the risk of heart disease, while omega-3 fats decrease it. Even saturated fats don't increase the risk of heart disease, if consumed in moderation as part of a healthy diet.

Coronary heart disease is still the leading cause of death in Australia. At the same time, the rate of obesity has exploded amongst children and adults since the 1980s, despite low-fat dietary guidelines, and despite the famous Heart Foundation tick that has been pointing to low fat products on our supermarket shelves for over 25 years.

The culprits seem to be sugar and trans fats, especially when these two ingredients are combined in manufactured products. Neither sugar nor fat on their own seem to be addictive, but when both are put together, the result is catastrophic! The sugar/fat combination, as in ice-cream, crisps and chocolate, affects the brain, as it stimulates your reward centre. When you eat these items, you experience a surge of *dopamine* in the brain, similar to what cocaine would give. These foods affect the brain in a way that natural products would never do.

Re-examine your relationship with fat. Instead of trying to eliminate it from your diet, be *aware* of it and keep your focus on *good* fats. One third of your calories should come from fat (hidden or in its pure form), so you don't need to deprive yourself of this essential nutrient. Eating fat increases your wellbeing and prevents cravings. Fat makes you feel fuller and less inclined to snack on high-calorie processed foods.

Today most people know it's better to avoid manufactured and takeaway foods, but these items are often convenient. The biggest and most popular fast food outlet in Australia is open 24 hours a day, and it's easy to drive through and grab something on your way.

Plan in advance and decide what you're going to eat before it's too late. Don't deviate from your intention. Don't feel guilty about eating fast food occasionally (e.g. once a month). But don't make it a habit, and avoid relying on it when you're hungry, as the nutritional value of these foods is questionable. They are basically empty calories, devoid of fibre and full of bad fats and sugar!

Maybe you believe that fat makes you fat, that you need to go on a low-fat diet if you want to lose weight. But fat is not the enemy. Fat is good for you, as long as you consume it thoughtfully: 20 to 35 % of your dietary intake should be from fat. So don't feel guilty if you enjoy your egg with the yolk, and your coffee with full cream milk!

Choose what sort of fats you will eat: good or bad. The bad ones are mainly found in highly processed foods and take away foods. They are trans fats, artificially created through hydrogenation of vegetable oils. This process makes them more suitable for the food industry. Trans fats enhance the texture, flavour and shelf life of many products, from cookies to frozen pizzas. Tantalizing your taste buds, they travel from your digestive system to your arteries, clogging them up by turning into a kind of thick, sticky paste that increases your heart and stroke risk.

Cooking or frying food in vegetable oil is a dangerous practice. When they're heated, the structure of these oils changes and they generate toxic compounds that increase the risk of degenerative diseases and cancer.

The belief that fat makes you fat probably derives from the fact that it is the macronutrient that has the most calories per gram. Fat contains 9 calories per gram, whereas carbohydrates and protein only contain 4 calories per gram. From a strictly caloric standpoint, it seems to make sense that fat is fattening. You will ingest too many calories if you have too much fat. But it is a simplistic view, and weight loss is not about calories alone. Fat is not just energy storage in the form of big thighs or a protruding belly!

Fat is *vitally* important for your health and survival:

- Fat is a structurally integral part of every single cell membrane in your body. We're not just talking fat cells. Every single cell in your body needs fat for every single function!

- Fat is needed to properly digest and assimilate the all-important fat-soluble vitamins A,D,E and K. Conveniently, many foods that contain these vitamins also have the fat required to digest them. The fat in the egg yolk allows the body to access the precious A and D vitamins so abundant in it. Milk is also rich in those vitamins and fat helps us absorb them. Fat is also needed to absorb calcium from milk. Skim milk is therefore not a good idea, as it lacks essential nutrients, or these nutrients cannot be assimilated.

- Fat is required for the adequate use of protein: egg whites won't help you, if you discard the valuable yolks with the fat in them!

- Fat is a powerful source of energy: a consistent, smooth-burning fuel that doesn't play havoc with your insulin and glucose metabolism. Fat is absorbed *slowly*, so the energy will last you longer.

- Fat slows sugar absorption, just like fibre does. Any sugar you eat enters the bloodstream more slowly in the presence of fat, which prevents your insulin from spiking. As a result, you'll be hungry *less* quickly. This is why ice cream has a lower GI (glycaemic index) than orange juice: the cream in it stops sugar from being absorbed too rapidly. Fat-free orange juice or jelly beans are often given to diabetics suffering a sudden drop in blow sugar. Orange juice and jelly beans have a very high GI, capable of raising blood sugar almost instantly. If you cut fat too low, you will be hungry, as your blood sugar will fluctuate. You will be tempted to snack and overeat, as you will experience more cravings.

- Fat adds flavour and texture to your food. Small amounts of oil, fresh butter or mayonnaise can make all the difference to a dish, by adding special interest and appeal to it.
- Fat plays an important role in regulating leptin and ghrelin, the hunger hormones. *Leptin* lets you know when you're full and it's time to expend energy while *ghrelin* (stomach growling!) accentuates your hunger feelings, and is particularly active just before a meal. Paradoxically, fat is good for weight loss because it suppresses ghrelin, the hormone that makes you want to eat. Without enough ghrelin, you're more likely to overeat.
- Fat plays a key role in managing inflammation. Some fats help your body inflame when it's useful, as a defence mechanism against infection, and other fats help your body *reduce* inflammation. Unfortunately, trans fats are in themselves highly inflammatory, because of the way they've been processed, and therefore damaging to the body.

There are four types of fat:

- Monounsaturated fat
- Polyunsaturated fat
- Saturated fat
- Trans fats

1) Monounsaturated and polyunsaturated fats are generally viewed as the 'good guys', as they seem to be beneficial for your heart, cholesterol, and overall health. They are also rich in omega 3 and omega 6 fatty acids, which are essential for your wellbeing.

- **Sources of monounsaturated fats:**

olive oil, canola oil, sunflower oil, peanut oil, sesame oil, avocados, olives, peanut butter and nuts (almonds, peanuts, pine nuts, macadamia nuts, hazelnuts, pecans, cashews).

- **Sources of polyunsaturated fats:**

soybean oil, corn oil, safflower oil, walnuts, sunflower, sesame and pumpkin seeds, flax seeds, soy milk, tofu and fatty fish (salmon, tuna, mackerel, herring, trout, sardines, shrimp). These foods are also rich in omega-3 fatty acids that are crucial to your health and that your body can't manufacture. You can only get these essential fatty acids from food sources and they support brain functions like memory and concentration, while reducing excessive inflammation in your body.

Our modern way of eating creates a deficit in omega 3, so it's important to ensure we're getting enough of it. Omega 3 fatty acids protect us from cardiovascular disease and enhance nerve and brain development and function. Contrary to popular belief, fish does not have the highest percentage of omega 3. Surprisingly, flax seeds and walnuts are the foods richest in omega 3. If you want your kids to be smart, give them walnuts. And a fascinating and amusing fact is that walnuts are shaped like brains!

2) Saturated fats also have health benefits and latest research has proven that they have basically *no* negative effect on blood cholesterol. Whole fat dairy products are a good source of calcium and protein, despite their high saturated fat content. Cold pressed *coconut oil* is a good energy and endurance booster. Eating saturated fats in moderation is advisable. Avoid cooking in fat and frying your food. Instead, add a bit of fat to your cooking when it's ready, like a drizzle of olive oil or a teaspoon of butter

or fresh cream. Pure and unadulterated coconut oil is the best cooking and frying oil.

- **Sources of saturated fats:**

Meats (beef, lamb, pork), chicken with the skin on, whole-fat dairy products (milk, yoghourt, cream, butter, cheese), egg yolk, palm and coconut oil.

Coconut oil has many health benefits. It is rich in a fatty acid called lauric acid, which can improve cholesterol and help kill bacteria and other pathogens. It is also ideal for high heat cooking, as it is very stable.

3) Trans fats, or hydrogenated oils, are the 'bad guys'. They are used in the food industry to help products remain consistent, retain freshness longer and make them more appealing to human consumption. Also called trans fatty acids, they put you at risk of cardiovascular disease, as they raise your low density lipoprotein or LDL cholesterol (bad cholesterol) and lower your high density lipoprotein or HDL cholesterol (good cholesterol).

These fats have been linked to insulin resistance, type 2 diabetes, as well as obesity, especially around the abdomen. Companies love using trans fatty acids as they are cheap, easy to make and convenient – perfect for packaged supermarket products and industrial bakery items, but not fit for humans.

- **Sources of trans fatty acids:**

French fries, anything deep fried or battered, pies and piecrust, margarine, shortening, cake mixes and frosting, pancake and waffle mix, fried chicken, ice cream, non-dairy creamers, microwave popcorn, ground beef, cookies, biscuits, frozen or creamy beverages, manufactured meat, crackers, frozen dinners,

Asian crunchy noodles, canned meals, packaged pudding, confectionery.

These foods taste good but are not good for you! It has been suggested that trans fats make junk food more addictive. This is true, especially when combined with sugar and salt. When you switch to a diet of clean, fresh foods you may even experience withdrawal symptoms for the first few days or week.

The problem with these fats is that your body doesn't quite know what to do with them. Your body can't break them down and use them correctly. Normal fats are supple and pliable, but trans fatty acids lack this flexibility. They are stiff and build up in your body where they create havoc and disturb normal processes. If you're serious about weight loss and keeping yourself healthy, you need to cut your consumption of these fats as low as possible: make them less than one percent of your total calories.

Fresh fruit, vegetables and legumes lower your cholesterol and help cleanse your body of trans fats along with other toxins. Always include them in your diet, and choose your fats carefully. Once all fats were judged unhealthy, and were made responsible for a myriad of diseases, from cardiovascular disease to diabetes and even cancer. But today experts agree that fats are an absolutely essential part of our diet.

There are different types of fats; some are good, and some are bad. The bad ones are the commercially produced fats found in convenience foods. Avoid these man-made fats as much as possible, especially in combination with sugar. Avoid cooking with fat, except for coconut oil. Focus on eating good fats, and have moderate amounts saturated fat from animal sources.

Key Points and Strategies:

- Don't think low fat, think good fat!
- One third of your calories should come from fat
- Eat monounsaturated and polyunsaturated fats – the 'good guys'. They come from vegetable products like olive oil, nuts and tofu, as well as fatty fish
- Don't use these oils for frying or cooking. Instead, drizzle olive oil over your dishes when ready
- Eat moderately of saturated fats from meat, poultry, egg yolk, full-cream dairy products and natural coconut oil (best cooking oil)
- Avoid at all costs trans fats – they are dangerous and addictive
- Eat a lot of fibre-rich foods like fruit, vegetables and beans to helps counteract the harmful effects of trans fats.

15

WATER – YOUR NATURAL FOUNTAIN OF YOUTH

Drinking water is a great way to detoxify your body and assist the function of all your tissues and organs. It also fills you up and helps you eat less!

Life originated deep beneath the surface of the ocean. Life came out of the water, and water is necessary for all life. At birth, water accounts for approximately 80 percent of an infant's body weight. Roughly 70 percent of an adult's body is made up of water. The human brain comprises about 85 percent water, and even your bones are not as hard as you think, as they are between 10 and 15 percent water.

While two-thirds of your body is made of water, every bodily function uses it too. We could go for several months without food, but, without water, we would only survive two or three days. This is because we can store fat, but, we can't store water. We might eat different foods in different parts of the world, but we all drink water. Water is not only the beginning of all life; it is the most essential nutrient of all, and it is the one we most take for granted.

Instead of having drinks containing sugar, caffeine, alcohol, milk or cream, quench your thirst with water. Water and is a major contributor to good health. Almost everyone has heard the advice: *Drink at least eight glasses of water a day*. This amounts to around two litres, considering a glass holds approximately 250 ml. You may not be able to eat as much as you want, but you can drink as much water as you like. Have one or two glasses of water as soon as you get out of bed: it will hydrate your skin and stimulate your metabolism and bowel function.

A point worth mentioning here: taking laxatives for weight loss is bad for you. Using them for a long period can cause serious health problems. When you take laxatives, water is drawn into the bowel to increase the bulk of your stool. Bowel muscles are stimulated to produce a motion. Any weight loss experienced while taking laxatives is attributed to water loss. The excretion of faecal matter gives your abdomen a flatter appearance, but this is only temporary. As soon as you eat and drink, any weight lost will return. This is because calories from food eaten are still absorbed in the small intestine. Taking laxatives does not reduce your caloric intake. Laxative abuse can cause dehydration, a lack in important nutrients, and electrolyte imbalance. Eventually, you'll be deficient in calcium, magnesium and potassium, which can have serious implications.

Laxatives are habit-forming. As your bowel becomes dependent on them and the muscles in your gut become weak, you will lose the ability to have a normal bowel movement without them. The result is rebound constipation! Daily laxative use or abuse with the intention of losing weight is symptomatic of an eating disorder. If you're genuinely constipated, it is safer is to drink plenty of water and eat lots of fibre.

You don't need to purchase expensive bottled water. Today, pollution is everywhere, in the ground, in the water and in the air. Even 'natural' spring water is not so natural any more, as it may be contaminated, even by the plastic bottle it's sold in. Purified tap water is an inexpensive alternative to bottled water, and a filter can extract chlorine and other harmful chemicals from your drinking water. Store your water in glass or stainless steel bottles, rather than plastic bottles, to prevent chemicals from leaching into it.

Twelve reasons why you should drink plenty of water every day:

1) For healthy, glowing skin.

Nothing improves the appearance of your complexion more than drinking water, as it moisturizes your skin from the inside out, and is much more effective than any expensive cream you can buy. It prevents your skin from drying out, thus reducing wrinkles and leaving it supple and elastic, with a beautiful shine.

2) To flush excess water and toxins from your body, while supporting liver and kidneys.

Without sufficient water, your body will go into *survival* mode and store excess water. When the body is supplied with a sufficient amount of water, it begins to release stores from your hips, thighs and ankles. Water helps remove these stores but also helps flush out waste products from your body by stimulating your kidneys. Water prevents the formation of kidney and bladder stones.

Water assists your liver function. Without enough water, the kidneys are unable to perform their function, which is filtering the blood and getting rid of toxins through urine. In the absence of sufficient water, the kidneys will turn to the liver for assistance.

The liver, which is a major 'rubbish' removal system, is then unable to perform some of its normal duties which include burning fat and calories. This results in the body depositing more fat. Water and fat stores going up means more weight on your body and on the scale.

An early sign of dehydration is headache, due to dehydrated brain cells, and an accumulation of toxins in the blood. You take Aspirin or Panadol, but it's the water you drink to swallow your tablets that actually corrects your headache.

3) Drinking at least eight glasses of water a day may reduce the risk of heart disease.

If your body lacks water, your heart will need to work harder in order to pump oxygenated blood towards your body cells, and there is a greater chance of fatigue and exhaustion, as well as damaging strain on your heart muscle.

4) Water cushions and lubricates your joints and muscles, thus enhancing performance during physical activity.

It also prevents muscle fatigue and pain, as well as cramps. It can also help with restless legs and contribute towards a good night's sleep, as it is a natural muscle relaxant.

5) Water gives you energy and helps you stay fit and alert with a positive mind.

You can face challenges more effectively when you drink water. Even minor levels of dehydration can cause headaches, drowsiness, moodiness, lack of concentration and lack of enthusiasm. The brain is for the most part made of water; logically, it will work better with it!

6) For optimal digestive function.

Water dilutes digestive juices in your stomach and prevents you from developing ulcers. During the passage of food in the gut, fibre absorbs water like a sponge, increasing bulk and softness of digested material. The end result is not difficult to imagine. When combined with a high fibre diet, water prevents constipation, without irritating the bowel like laxatives do. Laxatives are harmful, and using them regularly may cause *rebound* constipation. The bowel becomes lazy, as it loses its natural tone. Laxatives aggravate constipation, but water is a cheap cure without negative side effects.

7) Water strengthens your immune system.

It reduces the risk of contracting infectious and degenerative diseases. It even hampers the growth of abnormal and cancerous cells. Water has an overall *protective* effect on your health.

8) It regulates your body temperature, so you don't overheat.

When you have an elevated temperature, make sure you drink enough water to replace lost fluids. Water also assists sweating, which helps you cool down and conserve your energy.

9) Water makes you feel full and stimulates your metabolism, thus assisting weight loss.

Drinking water before a meal leaves less room for food. It reduces your appetite, and when you feel fuller, you're less likely to overeat. Water activates protein synthesis and muscle formation. It assists weight loss by encouraging the body to burn more calories, especially during exercise.

10) Water has healing properties.

When you're sick, it helps you recover quickly. It activates tissue regeneration and re-establishes a balance within all your systems. It helps alleviate vomiting and diarrhoea by replenishing water stores and preventing dehydration.

11) Drinking water helps prevent diabetes.

A lack of water inhibits insulin secretion and eventually leads to diabetes. Dehydration and diabetes go hand in hand. Thirst is not a reliable indicator: by the time you're thirsty, it's too late: you're already dehydrated! When your body doesn't get enough water, *histamine* becomes elevated, which causes your kidneys to release a special hormone that stops insulin from being produced. If you want to protect yourself against diabetes, increase your water consumption, and adhere to a gentle exercise program (e.g. walking for 30 minutes, four times a week).

12) Water has no calories, does not cause any weight gain, and it reduces fluid retention.

Due to mineral imbalances and overworked kidneys, an overweight body can retain a lot of water, which is why some people complain about *puffiness*. Once your fat starts melting and toxins leave your body, this bloating will disappear. Water assists this process, as it detoxifies your body. Perhaps you fear that too much water will make you feel waterlogged. The opposite is true, and unless you suffer from kidney disease, water does not increase oedema (swelling). On the contrary, it acts like a mild diuretic, increasing urine production.

Drinking water should be an essential part of your daily routine and diet plan. It will rev up your metabolism, accelerate weight loss and ward off health complications. Some people don't have a strong thirst sensation, but that doesn't mean they need to drink less. Drinking eight glasses of water a day is easy, inexpensive and it's one of the most powerful health boosters.

Some people complain that water tastes boring. Although H2O doesn't have a specific taste, it refreshes your palate and throat, which is a nice sensation. Some people find herbal tea more appealing. Be cautious with herbs, as not all of them are innocuous, and stick to the most common ones like mint or chamomile. A few drops of lemon juice can add zest to your water. Avoid lemonade, cordials and other soft drinks, as they contain a lot of sugar or artificial sugar, as well as additives.

Soft drinks are amongst the worst inventions of the twentieth century. They help overweight adults remain fat, and they are the cause of countless cases of obesity and tooth decay amongst children. Diet drinks containing artificial sweeteners are not recommended. Their long-term effects have not been researched properly, and some of them are thought to be responsible for serious health problems.

Thirst is often mistaken for hunger, but food doesn't quench your thirst; only water does. To cool yourself down you may have soft drinks, ice cream or flavoured yoghurt, but sugar will only make you thirstier. Caffeine (found in coffee, tea, cola and 'energy' drinks) and alcohol are not good thirst quenchers either, as they drain water and minerals from the body. Flavoured milks like chocolate, strawberry or banana milk are very high in sugar.

If you don't like water and are used to drinking sugary beverages, it will take some practice to switch to simple H2O. Water, the purest and most natural of all drinks, is much better for you, and it's also cheaper. To increase the amount of water you drink, start with one or two glasses in the morning, and have another one every hour or so.

People who drink a lot of water enjoy better health than those who don't. Drinking water, like breathing, is essential for life. Water is a fountain of youth and wellbeing available to everyone.

Key Points and Strategies:

- There are at least twelve health benefits associated with drinking water
- Water is good for weight loss, as it stimulates your metabolism and flushes toxins from your body
- Headache can be a sign of dehydration
- Make sure you drink at least eight glasses (two litres) of water a day
- Drink water before each meal to fill your stomach
- Use water as a natural laxative, in combination with a high-fibre diet
- Use water as a natural diuretic to reduce puffiness
- Don't have sugary drinks or artificially sweetened drinks
- Don't mistake thirst for hunger
- Continue to sip water throughout the day and you'll feel happier, more focused and more energetic.

16

PROTEIN: TOO MUCH OF A GOOD THING CAN BE HARMFUL

Eat animal protein in moderation for weight loss – and for health.

Protein is an integral part of a healthy diet. It promotes weight loss for different reasons. As well as helping you feel full, protein lowers *ghrelin,* the hormone that makes you hungry. Protein slows glucose absorption. By stabilizing your blood glucose levels, it gives you sustained energy throughout the day. Adding protein to your meal reduces its glycaemic impact. Glycaemic Index or GI ranks carbohydrates according to their effect on blood glucose level: the lower the GI, the slower the rise in blood glucose level. Your blood sugar is less likely to drop; you will be less hungry and experience cravings less frequently.

Proteins are the building blocks of life. In your body, they break down into *amino acids* that promote cell growth and repair. While every cell and organ in your body needs protein, consuming too much protein can be harmful. Excessive protein causes toxins to build up in your bloodstream, which can prevent your organs from functioning properly, and which can ultimately lead to permanent damage. Protein should make up no more than 10 to 35 % of your total caloric intake. Physically active people need more protein than sedentary individuals.

Dr Atkins promoted a high protein, high fat and low carb diet. For over 40 years, Dr Atkins' *Diet Revolution* and *New Diet Revolution* sold like hot cakes. Dr Atkins died in 2003 at the age of 72, but not of a heart condition like some people viciously rumoured. While on his way to work, he slipped on icy pavement and smashed his head. **Dr Atkins low-carb, high fat diet gained a huge following and today, m**any people still believe carbohydrates are fattening. They believe you need to follow a high-protein diet to lose weight, even though there is enough scientific evidence that this can be detrimental to your health.

Eight reasons why high-protein diets are bad for weight loss *and* your health:

1) Bone loss and osteoporosis, especially in women.

High-protein diets have been shown to work for weight loss, at least in the beginning. But protein (specifically *animal* protein) contains *acid,* which is potentially harmful. Animal protein affects your bone density when eaten in large amounts. Scientists found that women who ate more meat than vegetable protein had a higher incidence of bone loss and hip fractures than women who eat both types of protein. Due to their calcium content, your bones help neutralize excess acid in your body. Kidneys excrete acid in your urine, but as you get older, your kidneys become less efficient. To compensate, bones become involved in neutralizing acid. Fruit and vegetables can also help restore the body's PH balance and create a more alkaline environment. Excess animal protein leaches calcium from your bones, making your skeleton more brittle and fragile. It also reduces the body's ability to absorb calcium. This happen after just six weeks on a high-protein diet!

2) Kidney stones.

The popularity of high-protein diets has created a rise in the incidence of kidney stones. The acidic environment produced by animal protein increases the formation of these crystals, while plant protein doesn't have the same effect. Researchers found that six weeks on a low carbohydrate, high-protein diet considerably increases the load to the kidneys. Animal protein has been shown to boost urinary excretion of *oxalate*, a compound that combines with calcium and other compounds. Together they form kidney stones. Fruit and vegetables have a protective effect as they are high in potassium, which helps ward off kidney stones.

3) Weight gain.

With carbs having such a bad reputation, many people would rather eat protein, as it builds muscle and seems to have more health benefits. Carbs and protein both have four calories per gram: they are equal from a caloric standpoint. But your body can only use a certain amount of protein each day, while the rest is stored as fat. Carbohydrate is the body's preferred fuel and calories from complex carbs will be used up during daily activities. Foods high in animal protein often contain substantial amounts of fat, which has nine calories per gram. Many people think protein is better than carbohydrates. They tend to eat more animal protein without being aware of the dangers. This can lead to weight gain as well as other unwanted effects.

4) Heart disease.

Too much animal protein makes you prone to heart disease. Protein often comes with fat, so you tend to consume more animal fat than if you were to follow a diet based on carbs and vegetable protein. High-protein diets contain less vitamins and antioxidants capable of preventing heart disease. They generally lack fibre, which is essential to maintain healthy blood cholesterol and a healthy heart. A healthy animal protein is *chicken breast*, while a healthy vegetable protein is *broccoli,* for instance. Chicken breast mainly consists of protein and fat. And while broccoli may not contain as much protein, it also offers fibre, vitamins, minerals and other essential nutrients that will keep you in good shape.

5) Ketosis.

When you eat too much protein and not enough carbohydrates, your body goes into *ketosis.* Your body starts using fat for energy instead of glucose. This may sound good but in reality it isn't. When fat is broken down it produces ketones, which are poisonous and cause an array of health problems. Your body will eliminate these ketones through your urine, as long as you drink enough water. Ketosis can quickly dehydrate you, by leaching fluid from your body. Your kidneys and liver suffer as they have to work overtime. Ketosis can impair your liver function and slow your metabolism. When your liver is busy removing excessive toxins from your body, there is not enough time to burn fat. Symptoms of ketosis are fatigue, headache, dizziness, heart palpitations and bad breath. It puts a lot of stress on your heart, while muscle mass and bone mass both decline as a result.

6) Reduced liver and brain function.

While too much protein harms your liver, which is your major detoxification organ, it can also affect your brain and nervous system. When you eat animal protein, your body produces *ammonia,* which is a toxin that your liver needs to process. If you eat too much protein over a period of time, your liver will be overworked. Ammonia and other damaging substances will build up in your bloodstream, which may lead to encephalopathy. This is a condition marked by a decline of brain and nervous system function. Your ability to focus and be attentive, to process and retain information, will be affected. You will feel lethargic, moody and depressed. Ultimately, your overall health and fitness will deteriorate.

7) Cancer, arthritis and gout.

All animal protein is acidic. Cancer cells thrive in an acidic environment, but are less likely to survive in an alkaline body. High-protein and high-fat diets also contribute to the development of *osteoarthritis.* These diets thicken your blood and harden your arteries, slowing and restricting the blood flow to your extremities, as well as to your bones and joints. Joint tissue degenerates and becomes less flexible, resulting in stiff and painful joints. *Gout* is a form of arthritis caused by the build-up of uric acid crystals in the joints. Uric acid comes from the breakdown of substances called purines. Animal proteins are high in purines, which can lead to an overproduction of uric acid that the kidneys struggle to eliminate. As a result, uric acid crystals form and accumulate in the joints where they cause swelling and inflammation.

8) Constipation, diverticulitis and bowel cancer.

When you increase your animal protein intake, you tend to eat less fibre-rich foods such as fruit, vegetables, whole grains, legumes, nuts and seeds. The result is *constipation.* Excessive animal protein creates an imbalance in your gut flora, reducing the number of 'friendly' bacteria. Your stool will smell horribly foul and may be hard to pass. You may also have alternative bouts of diarrhoea and constipation. Lack of fibre slows intestinal motility or peristalsis. Your stool will remain in your gut for much longer than necessary, releasing harmful toxins into your bloodstream. Not drinking enough water makes constipation worse, as your faeces become dry, compact and hard to expel.

Diverticulitis is a painful inflammation of the small outpouchings along the wall of the colon or large intestine. It is preceded by *diverticulosis*, the formation of these pouches due to a weakening of the colon walls. A key factor in the development of diverticulosis is elevated pressure within the colon. This pressure is raised when a person is compelled to push in order to pass hard bits of stool ('rabbit droppings').

Chronic constipation makes you feel bloated, headachy and irritable. According to scientific studies, it also puts you at risk of developing *bowel cancer*. A diet high in animal products, especially red meat and processed meats, has been directly associated with bowel cancer.

Animal-based foods such as beef, chicken, pork, lamb, fish and seafood are sometimes called 'complete' proteins, as they contain all the amino acids you need. 'Incomplete' proteins contain some, but not all, of these essential amino acids. Incomplete proteins are found in plant-based foods such as grains, legumes, seeds and nuts. It was believed that you needed to eat several foods containing incomplete proteins in each meal, to make up for the lack of certain essential amino acids in plant-based foods. But research has shown that incomplete protein foods can be eaten separately at any time. In combination, they will provide all the amino acids your body requires to function properly.

Vegetable protein is not inferior to animal protein. Plant foods, besides supplying good quality protein, provide other nutrients that have a protective effect against diseases; e.g., antioxidants, plant phenols, vitamins and minerals, soluble and insoluble fibre.

Nine vegetable protein-laden 'super foods':

1) Green peas

These humble little guys tend to be underestimated, probably because they're ubiquitous and cheap. But they're packed with protein, fibre and complex carbohydrates, as well as antioxidant and anti-inflammatory phytonutrients. One of them, a polyphenol called *coumestrol,* has a protective effect against stomach cancer. Although low in fat, peas are rich in omega 3 and omega 6 fatty acids and are a good source of vitamin E, which helps prevent coronary heart disease. Extremely versatile, frozen peas are okay for convenience, as long as they've only been frozen once. However, nothing compares to the flavour of fresh, shelled peas. Peas are easy-peasy to grow if you have a veggie patch!

2) Beans, lentils and chick peas

Unassuming, inexpensive, environmentally friendly and rich in protein, legumes are the ultimate key to permanent weight loss and wellbeing. Beans are full of *antioxidants*; lentils are a well-known source of *iron,* and chick peas contain a unique kind of fibre that has a protective effect against colon cancer. Legumes cleanse your liver, assist your kidneys and protect your heart. They also stabilise your blood sugar levels, thus preventing type 2 diabetes. They can be turned into loaves, breads, burgers, cakes, cookies, pancakes, patties, pies, puddings, muffins, mash, fudge, fritters, soups, stews, salads, dahl, curries, casseroles, hummus, spreads, quiches, tortillas, burritos, tacos... Check out the internet for thousands of mouth-watering recipes. There are so many ways to turn legumes into the most delicious plant-based dishes!

3) Tofu and tempeh

Tofu (or soybean curd) originated in China. It results from grinding soybeans into a milk-like substance, which is then compressed and left to coagulate. After the mass has dried into a gelatinous solid, it is cut into rectangular cubes the size of your hand. This rectangle is then cut into smaller, bite-sized cubes, ready for cooking or adding to salads.

Tempeh, a traditional soy product originally from Indonesia, is made by a natural culturing and controlled fermentation process that binds soy beans into a cake form.

Both tofu and tempeh are extremely versatile, and have a wide array of textures and uses. Your imagination is the only limit to what you can do with these fabulous, great-tasting vegetable protein foods. Visit the internet for thousands of tempting images and recipes.

Tofu and tempeh are perfect plant proteins, as they provide all eight essential amino acids, as well as being a good source of iron, calcium, vitamin B and folate (naturally occurring form of folic acid). Anything made from soy beans is a perfect protein. There is a misconception that vegetarians don't get as much protein as meat eaters do. The only difference between tofu and meat protein is that you need to have more tofu to achieve the recommended protein levels. Every 100 g of firm tofu yields about 12 g of protein, whereas 100 g of beef has 26 g. You would have to eat twice as much tofu to ingest the same amount of protein; without the extra fat and calories, as tofu is very low in both and contains no animal fat. But even without meat or dairy products, tofu would not be your sole source of protein, as you would include whole grains, legumes, seeds and nuts in your diet.

When consumed regularly instead of meat, tofu reduces your total cholesterol, triglycerides and low-density lipoprotein (bad cholesterol), as well as lowering your blood pressure. Rich in *isoflavones* that have powerful antioxidant properties, tofu protects your cells from damage caused by free radicals. Tofu prevents breast cancer, as evidenced by a study of Japanese women. Those who had the highest consumption of tofu had the lowest rates of breast cancer. In Asian nations that have soy-heavy diets, prostate cancer is far less common than in Australia, where we eat little soy. Tofu is known to alleviate premenstrual syndrome as well as menopause symptoms. It prevents osteoporosis by making middle-aged bones stronger.

4) Quinoa

Used by the Incas in the Andes as a staple food for 5000 years, and referred to as the 'mother seed', this ancient, highly nutritious gluten-free grain (which is actually a type of seed) is packed with health and healing properties. Low in calories, it contains more protein than any other grain (14 g of protein for 100 g of uncooked quinoa), with a good balance of all eight essential amino acids. It is high in fibre and has a low GI, ideal for keeping blood sugar levels stable. Quinoa is a good source of iron, B vitamins, calcium and magnesium. It is *alkaline*-forming, thus keeping in check the acid environment propitious to many diseases including cancer.

Quinoa is coated with toxic plant chemicals called saponins, so it's important to rinse it well. These compounds are used to promote healing of skin injuries in South America. There are three main varieties of quinoa: white or sweet, red, and black. Quinoa has a fluffy consistency and a nutty flavour. With this super food, moderation is the key: it shouldn't be consumed more often than two or three times a week. There are endless recipes with quinoa: tabouleh-style salads, chilies, stew, curries, desserts, stuffed vegetables, soups, stir fries, burgers, patties, loaves, porridge, pudding, biscuits, cakes, falafels and burritos.

5) Chia

Salvia hispanica, commonly known as chia, is a species of flowering plant in the mint family, native to central and southern Mexico, as well as Guatemala. Cultivated by the Aztecs and Mayans since around 3500 BC, chia seeds were considered magical for their ability to increase stamina and long-lasting energy. A complete protein with all eight essential amino acids, chia is high in complex carbohydrates and loaded with vitamins, minerals and antioxidants.

Each 100g of chia seeds provides:

- more protein than eggs
- more omega 3 fatty acids than salmon
- more fibre than oats
- more calcium than milk.

Chia seeds can be used as an egg substitute, to make healthy puddings and ice-creams, to thicken soups or gravies, to make grain-free crackers or biscuits, to thicken meatballs instead of using bread crumbs. They can be sprouted for salads, sprinkled over breakfast cereal or yoghurt, turned into smoothies and muesli bars. They can be eaten by themselves: a couple of tablespoons on the go will leave you surprisingly full. They do stick to your teeth though, but you can wash them down with some water or herbal infusion.

6) Nuts: almonds, walnuts, pecans, cashews, pistachios, brazil nuts, hazelnuts, macadamia nuts, pine nuts and peanuts

These small dry fruit with hard shells grow on trees or bushes. Inside the shell, the edible kernel is also called a *nut.* Peanuts are actually legumes, but are referred to as 'nuts', as they share many characteristics with tree nuts. Nuts are incredibly rich in protein:

100g of peanuts yield 26g of protein: the equivalent of 100g of beef! 100g of almonds yield 21 g of protein.

Research shows that people who eat nuts as a part of a weight loss diet show greater weight reduction than those who don't. Nuts stabilise your blood sugar levels, keeping hunger and cravings at bay. They promote the release of the hormone *leptin* in the gut, which promotes a feeling of satiety and fullness, while increasing energy expenditure.

Nuts are high in fat, but it is 'good' fat. They mainly contain healthy monounsaturated and polyunsaturated fats that don't clog up your arteries. Nuts lower your cholesterol, guarding against arteriosclerosis, high blood pressure and heart disease. Full of valuable nutrients, nuts will enhance any diet, but they are particularly important for vegetarians and vegans as a meat substitute.

Rich in fibre, complex carbohydrates, valuable antioxidants, vitamins (especially folate, vitamin B6 and vitamin E) and minerals (including calcium, iron, magnesium, zinc, copper and selenium), nuts complete a well-rounded diet and are known to increase your longevity. This is partly because they are high in omega 3 as well as anti-cancer compounds. Omega 3 assists your immune system and improves skin conditions. It helps reduce swelling and inflammation in your joints if you have arthritis. This fatty acid supports your nervous system and enhances brain function: memory and cognition. Nuts have been shown to prevent Alzheimer's disease, possibly due to the combination of omega 3, folate and vitamin E. Each variety of nuts has unique properties.

→ **Almonds** are ideal for dieters, as they are highly nutritious but low in calories. They also have *probiotic* properties: regular consumption of these nuts improves digestion, reduces the number of 'bad' bacteria in the gut, prevents constipation and accelerates your metabolism. Try almond milk instead of soy as a delicious and nutritious dairy milk alternative.

→ **Peanuts** contain *resveratrol*, a special antioxidant also found in grapes, red wine and grape juice. It is not concentrated in the skin as in grapes, but in the nut itself. Resveratrol prevents heart disease, cancer, diabetes, premature ageing and Alzheimer's disease.

→ **Pine nuts** contain *pinolenic acid*, which curbs your appetite and helps you lose or maintain your weight.

→ **Brazil nuts** are very high in *selenium* which has anti-cancer properties. Too much selenium can be toxic though, so be cautious and stick to one or two Brazil nuts a day, or a handful per week.

Due to their high fat and calorie content, as well as their powerful health properties, nuts should be consumed in moderation. A handful a day is the recommended amount, which amounts to about 30 almonds or ten whole walnuts.

7) 'Open Sesame': the magical food

Just like nuts, sesame seeds are high in protein and packed with nutrients: vitamins, minerals and valuable monounsaturated fatty acids. Sesame is a magical food, due to its medicinal and healing properties. It's is one of the oldest cultivated plants in the world and its history as a medicine date back to Ancient Egypt, 3500 BC. In Ancient Babylon, up to 600 BC, women used a mixture of honey and sesame paste (tahini) to preserve their youth and beauty, both internally as a supplement, and externally as a face mask. In the Roman Empire, soldiers ate the same mixture for strength and stamina.

There is now scientific evidence that sesame has numerous health enhancing properties. It lowers blood sugar, thus being helpful in the prevention and treatment of type 2 diabetes. It is beneficial for your heart and against stroke, as it prevents arteriosclerosis and lowers blood pressure when consumed regularly. Sesame has a protective effect against neurodegenerative diseases such as Alzheimer's, Parkinson's and multiple sclerosis. Due to its natural *antibiotic* properties, sesame oil helps reduce plaque, tooth decay and gingivitis when used as a mouth wash, by swirling it around in your mouth.

Other seeds packed with protein, fibre, calcium, iron, magnesium, vitamins and omega 3 fatty acids include hemp seeds, pumpkin seeds, sunflower seeds, flax seeds, cumin seeds, grape seeds, pomegranate seeds and apricot seeds. Each of them has special nutritional and medicinal properties, so make this living food an integral part of your diet for improved health and vitality!

8) Leafy green vegetables

Greens are the number one food to eat regularly in order to improve your health and wellbeing. Leafy greens are generally not high in protein compared to other foods, but they have so many health benefits that it's worth including them in your diet every day. Some greens are richer in protein than others. For instance, cooked broccoli contains 4 g of protein per cup, which is not negligible. A cup of cooked spinach yields 5 g, while a cup of Brussels sprouts will give you 4 g. And of course green peas are the champions, with almost 8 g of protein for a single cup!

9) Wheat meat or wheat gluten, also called seitan

This Japanese meat substitute made from gluten, the main protein of wheat is produced by washing wheat flour dough with water until all the starch granules are removed. The elastic mass of insoluble gluten is then cooked and eaten. Seitan is the vegetarian answer to roast beef. . You can simply chop up your seitan and add it to your carbs and vegetables to make a delicious meal. Or try fried seitan with capsicum (peppers) and onions served with brown rice or quinoa, and topped with sesame seeds.

Supermarkets carry an array of great tasting vegetarian and vegan options like veggie burgers, vegetarian sausages and meat-free minced meat, as well as vegetarian 'meat' pies, sausage rolls, fake bacon, and chicken-free chicken patties. These products use wheat gluten as their main ingredient. They are easily mistaken for the real stuff. I routinely use a wheat gluten-based minced meat in my lasagne and my children never guess they're eating a vegetarian meal! If you're allergic to wheat or gluten, seitan is a no-no of course, but it can be a good choice for people who are allergic to soy, nuts or certain legumes.

The importance of protein in your diet cannot be emphasised enough. A constant urge to eat refined carbs and sugary snacks can be a sign that you're lacking protein. However, you don't need to eat more chicken or beef to correct this symptom. You can increase your vegetable protein intake by adding some super foods to your daily intake. A lack of protein can also be responsible for low energy levels. If you get tired easily, try a vegan protein powder-shake to complement your breakfast and lunch. It will stop your blood sugar from fluctuating and will help you stay alert throughout your day, as well as warding off cravings.

Red meat is traditionally a 'male' food. Men often refuse to give up red meat or reduce their intake, claiming that they need it to function, as well as to build muscle and stamina. This attitude is deeply rooted in our culture and is related to gender identity. Eating meat is part of the tough male image that the media promotes. In an age of high technology, traditional rites of passage have become fuzzy or inexistent. There is no clear marker any more for the transition of boy to manhood. Males seem to yearn for a period when things were simpler and more evident, and some would like to go back as far as pre-historic times! To them, eating red meat is part of being a hunter or a warrior: a 'real' man. Our ancestors were hunters and ate meat, although not in quantities as large as we do today. But they were also mainly gatherers and the bulk of their diet consisted of wild fruit and veggies, as these were a more reliable source of nourishment.

Our bodies are not capable of manufacturing vitamin C, as we have evolved to eat primarily fresh plant foods. In that respect humans are unlike carnivores, who are capable of manufacturing their own vitamin C and therefore don't need fresh fruit or veggies to survive. Throughout history, males have not always insisted on eating meat. Roman soldiers would complain when given too much meat, and request more carbohydrates for energy during battle. While it is true that males have an overall greater need for protein than women (their overall caloric need is also greater), they can easily obtain protein from plant-based sources.

A widespread myth is that you need extra protein to build muscle. But even the protein powder manufacturers haven't been able to prove that there is a correlation between more protein and more muscle, once the minimum required amount is met. As long as you get the minimum required, eating more protein on top of that has virtually *no* effect besides the extra calories. Studies have shown that you will gain significantly more muscle by getting extra calories from complex carbohydrates. What really builds muscle tissue is not protein, but *exercise.* The more you use your muscles, the stronger they become.

Many superstar male athletes and role models are vegetarian or vegan, and they certainly don't suffer a lack of muscle mass or male strength: e.g. Robert Parish, Prince Fielder, Day Scott, Carl Lewis, Robert Cheeke, Mac Danzig, Mike Tyson, Brendon Brazier, Jake Shields, Rip Esselstyn, Georges Laraque and Michael Clarke Duncan just to name a few. If you would like more information on this subject as well as other interesting topics, there are many inspiring documentaries on YouTube, such as 'Plant-strong & healthy living' by Rip Esselstyn at TEDxFremont, and 'Debunking the paleo diet' by Christina Warinner at TEDxOU.

A lack of red meat has been blamed for anaemia. Iron-deficiency anaemia is a condition caused by insufficient dietary intake and absorption of iron. It affects women more than men, due to blood loss during menstruation. Iron is essential for blood production, and thus for providing energy for daily activities. About two thirds of your body's iron is found in the red blood cells of your blood, in the form of *haemoglobin*.

Haemoglobin is a red protein responsible for the transport of oxygen in your blood. Without iron, the body can't synthesise haemoglobin. Symptoms of anaemia are fatigue, pale skin (or paleness in the lining of the eyes and mouth), weakness, shortness of breath, headaches, frequent infections, dizziness or light-headedness, cold hands and feet, fast heartbeat, brittle nails, and sometimes weird cravings. Traditionally, red meat is recommended for its iron content, but it's not the only source of this important mineral.

- → **Mussels:** one of the best sources of iron. Twenty small mussels contain 15 mg of iron, as well as being high in selenium and vitamin B12
- → **Oysters:** twelve oysters have 7 mg of iron, as well as being rich in zinc and low in calories;
- → **Steak:** a 150 mg steak has 5.55 mg of iron
- → **Eggs:** two large eggs have 2 mg of iron
- → **Silver beet**: one cup of cooked silver beet has 2.53 mg of iron
- → **Cashews:** 30 g contain 1.5 mg of iron
- → **Prune juice:** one cup contains 3.15 mg of iron, as well as being a natural remedy for constipation.

The recommended daily intake of iron for women aged 19 to 50 is 18 mg a day. For men it is only 8 mg. Overloading the body with iron is dangerous, as excess iron accumulates in the liver and may cause serious complications such as cirrhosis, diabetes and heart problems. This is why eating too much red meat can be bad for you. Red meat has also been linked to coronary heart disease and stroke, due to its *carnitine* content, as well as to diabetes and cancer. 'Eating red meat increases the risk of dying early' says Dr Adam Bernstein, research director at the U.S. Cleveland Clinic's Wellness Institute, and co-author of a 28 –year study on red meat and life expectancy.

To absorb iron from your diet, you need vitamin C. As the body can't manufacture its own vitamin C, you need to eat vitamin C rich foods every day. Rather than eating more red meat, eat more fresh fruit and raw vegetables; their high content of vitamin C will help you absorb iron from your food, especially from plant sources like legumes or whole grains.

Dairy products are a good source of protein and calcium. Just as iron is often linked to red meat, calcium is traditionally associated with milk and dairy products. Calcium, the most abundant mineral in the body, is vital for strong bones and teeth. It also helps the body maintain healthy blood vessels, regulates blood pressure and even prevents insulin resistance (a precursor of type 2 diabetes). The recommended daily calcium intake is 1000 mg for women aged 19 to 50, which can be found in roughly three serves of dairy (one serve = a cup of milk or a thick slice of cheddar cheese). With allergies on the rise and many people being lactose intolerant, milk alternatives like soy, almond, oat milk or rice milk have become popular. These products are often calcium-fortified, which puts them on par with dairy milk.

There are many other sources of calcium apart from dairy: leafy greens, seafood, legumes, nuts, seeds, and fruit (oranges and cranberries in particular). Calcium requires the presence of vitamin D to be absorbed. The most natural way to get vitamin D is to expose your bare skin to the sunlight (ultraviolet B rays). This can work quickly in the Australian summer. The amount of sunshine needed depends on how fair your skin is. It ranges from ten minutes for a very light-skinned individual, up to a couple of hours for a darker skinned person. The more skin revealed, the better the effect. You can also get vitamin D from a limited range of food sources. It occurs naturally in cod liver oil, fatty fish like salmon, tuna or mackerel, oysters, caviar (fish eggs) and mushrooms. A lot of products such as breakfast cereals, orange juice, dairy and soy products are fortified with this important vitamin.

Calcium works in conjunction with magnesium. This essential mineral is found in dark leafy greens such as raw spinach, nuts and seeds (especially pumpkin seeds), fish (mackerel), beans and lentils, whole grains, avocados, bananas and dates (the fruit, not the romantic appointment). A craving for chocolate may be a sin or sign of a magnesium-poor diet, as chocolate has very high levels of magnesium; nevertheless, chocolate needs to be consumed in moderation due to its sugar content. It is safer to increase the amount of legumes, nuts and seeds you eat, as these are also naturally high in calcium. Magnesium is the key to the body's proper assimilation of calcium and vitamin D.

Dr Carolyn Dean, author of the book *The Magnesium Miracle*, says that, without adequate levels of magnesium, the effectiveness and benefits of calcium regarding bone health and the prevention of osteoporosis are enormously impaired. Excess calcium actually becomes toxic in the absence of magnesium, and may contribute to arthritis, kidney stones, osteoporosis, as well as calcification of the arteries leading to high blood pressure and coronary heart disease.

A lot of foods are naturally rich in calcium, so you don't have to drink large quantities of dairy milk to get enough of it. Western countries are the biggest consumers of dairy products but we also have the highest rate of osteoporosis. In Australia, over one in five women over the age of 65 have osteoporosis, which means they have lost more than half of their bone density. This disease which leads to fragile bones, deformities and fractures, is caused by a number of factors, the most important of which is excess animal protein. This is not an area of controversy, as it is evidenced and supported by scientific research.

The link between excess animal protein intake and bone loss is direct and consistent. Even with a very high calcium intake, the more excess animal protein in the diet, the greater the incidence of negative calcium balance, and the greater the loss of calcium from your bones. Dr John McDougall, a leading medical authority on the subject, recommends that the most important dietary change we can make if we want to create a positive calcium balance that will keep our bones solid is to decrease the amount of animal protein we eat.

Excess animal protein contributes to an acidic environment, which depletes your bones. The body has to 'steal' alkalising minerals such as calcium from the skeleton to keep the blood from dropping into the acid range (normally, your blood maintains a slightly alkaline range). Other factors may also increase your risk of osteoporosis: excess dietary salt, excess alcohol consumption, nicotine, caffeine and a lack of exercise – in particular, weight-bearing exercise.

Key Points and Strategies:

- Don't focus on high-protein. Instead, think *less* animal and *more* vegetable protein

- Eat moderate amounts of chicken, red meat and seafood as part of a healthy diet
- Include whole grains, legumes, seeds and nuts in your daily diet for vegetable protein
- Be aware that consuming excess animal protein can increase your risk of osteoporosis, heart disease and other health problems
- 'Super foods' like *chia* contain high quality plant-based protein, as well as numerous other health-enhancing properties that will boost your vitality and support your weight loss effort
- Men don't need more meat than women
- Red meat is not your only source of iron and there are other iron-rich foods, like mussels and prune juice
- Increase your *vitamin C* intake (found in fresh fruit and veggies) to absorb iron from your diet
- Dairy products are rich in protein and calcium but can cause allergies. Use them in moderation and consider milk alternatives like soy or almond milk
- There are other sources of calcium besides cow's milk, like legumes, nuts, seeds and seafood (these are also rich in magnesium)
- Vitamin D is important to absorb calcium from your diet. You can obtain it from sunlight or food sources, especially fortified products
- Magnesium is the *key* to calcium uptake in the body.

17

SUGAR AND SPICE AND ALL THINGS NICE

Eat less sugar and your weight will drop.

The only good thing about sugar is that it tastes nice. It's tempting to say 'Don't ever eat sugar again', but you probably enjoy the occasional sweet indulgence. Be aware of what sugar does to you if you consume it excessively. Reduce your intake, especially in the form of soft drinks (sodas), processed supermarket foods and take-away foods. You don't need to cut it out of your diet completely. Sugar is potentially harmful, and some people have managed to quit it altogether. But what may even be more harmful is a negative attitude to life!

Studies have shown that a happy person with a positive attitude to life will have better health than someone with a negative attitude. This is true even when the positive person has some unhealthy lifestyle habits. Happiness results in higher serotonin and endorphin levels. These feel-good hormones are satisfying, so you tend *not* to crave sugar.

A diet rich in complex carbohydrates can increase serotonin levels in the brain. It prevents you from being hungry and turning to sugary treats. Also include vegetable protein in your meals, and you'll crave these high-calorie killers even less. Fruit is a good snack, rich in fibre, which slows the absorption of natural sugar.

Sugar is addictive, and it acts like a *painkiller* in the body, for both physical and emotional pain. Some individuals are more susceptible to this effect than others. Some experts claim that sugar can be eight times more addictive than heroin. This is bad news if you're overweight or obese. A period of detox might be necessary: going cold turkey or cutting down your sugar intake progressively.

I must emphasise that, when you quit an addiction, you need to replace it with something else. Think about what you can do to relax and enjoy life without sugar. Reduce stress and learn how to meditate, emptying your mind or focusing on a positive quote. Louise L. Hay publishes daily affirmations on her website louisehay.com. There are numerous other websites that will deliver daily positive messages to your email.

For over 30 years we thought fat was the dietary evil, but Dr Robert Lustig proves us wrong. He pioneered a war against sugar: he brands it as *toxic* and *poisonous*, especially in the way it is consumed today. It's not sweet any more: it's a killer. Due to evolution, we are programmed to love anything that tastes sweet, as it means that it is safe for us to eat. In nature, fructose is contained in small amounts in fruits. But we can't eat too much fruit at once (who can eat ten apples or oranges?) and fibre slows the absorption of its sugar. Fruit juice is a concentrated form of fruit without the fibre. If you decide to include it in your diet, stick to a small glass a day (150 ml).

High fructose corn syrup is a concentrated form of sugar, which is added to numerous processed foods and beverages, including items that don't normally taste sweet, like soups or sauces. Dr Robert Lustig blames high fructose corn syrup for the obesity epidemic. He believes it is responsible for the increase in type 2 diabetes, hypertension, stroke, heart disease, Alzheimer's disease, and possibly even cancer. When you consume too much fructose, the liver is overloaded and turns the excess into fat. This fat reaches the bloodstream in the form of LDL (bad cholesterol) and is then deposited on the walls of your arteries, causing them to harden and narrow. If you ingest too much fructose, tiny fat droplets will begin to accumulate in your liver cells. This build-up is called non-alcoholic fatty liver disease, as it replicates what happens in the livers of people who drink too much alcohol. At the same time, there is a build-up of fat around your organs (visceral fat), leading to abdominal obesity or 'having an apple shape': one of the characteristics of *metabolic syndrome.*

Limiting sugar in your diet is one of the keys to longevity. Of all the molecules capable of inflicting damage in your body, sugar molecules are probably the most harmful. Fructose is a potent pro-inflammatory agent that speeds up ageing. Glycation is a process in which sugar attaches itself to proteins in your blood to form new molecules. These new molecules, called 'advanced glycation end products' or 'AGEs' (an appropriate acronym), are *destructive* to adjacent proteins. Most vulnerable to damage are collagen and elastin, the protein fibres that keep your skin firm and elastic. AGEs make your skin more prone to sagging and wrinkling, so avoid sugar if you want to preserve a youthful appearance!

From the early seventies to the mid-nineties, we were advised to reduce our fat intake to prevent coronary heart disease. But without fat, food doesn't taste nice. As a result, the food industry replaced fat with sugar, as it was believed to be a better choice.

Eating low-fat flavoured yoghurt is almost the equivalent of eating candy! Sugar causes a spike in insulin followed by rebound low blood sugar: you will crave more sugar shortly after eating it. Sugar stimulates pleasure centres in the brain, producing a *euphoric* effect, just like alcohol or drugs do. You can even build up a tolerance: the more sugar you eat, the less you'll feel the effect from it, so you need to increase your intake all the time.

Robert Lustig says it's essential that we limit our sugar intake to no more than 150 calories from sugar for men and 100 calories from sugar for women. This is less than the total sugar contained in a can of soft drink (soda). Many foods high in sugar are also high in fat, especially trans fats, such as ready-made cakes, sweet biscuits, cookie mixes and chocolate bars, which is another reason to avoid them. Today, processed food is without doubt the most damaging aspect of most people's diet, contributing to excess weight, poor health and chronic disease, and this is due to its fructose and trans fat content.

Artificial sweeteners are not recommended:

- They are manufactured products, just like their name implies, usually made from chemicals
- They may increase your appetite by stimulating your taste buds and hunger centres in your brain.
- They may increase insulin production, leading to low blood sugar, weakness and cravings.
- *Aspartame* (NutraSweet or Equal) is a chemical sweetener commonly used in sugar-free products, with many reported serious side effects, ranging from migraine headaches to hallucinations, seizures and brain tumors. It's not worth consuming it for the sake of saving a few calories.
- *Sucralose* (Splenda) is just as scary: it may enlarge both liver and kidneys, and shrink the thymus gland. Splenda

can cause skin rashes, panic attacks, diarrhoea, headaches, bladder problems, and stomach pains.

- Studies have shown that artificial sweeteners can cause overeating in those who consume them.

Wean yourself off the sweet taste gradually, until you don't crave it any more. Drink *water* every time you long for a can of soft drink. Eat *fruit* instead of candy or cookies. Sugar is a habit, not a necessity. If you insist on using a low-calorie sugar substitute, I would recommend STEVIA, a natural product made from the leaves of a shrub native to Paraguay and Brazil, where it has been used for hundreds of years, mainly for its medicinal properties. Don't use stevia in large amounts though, as it could cause unknown side effects and could interact with certain pharmaceuticals.

Sugar is an addictive substance with a strong psychological component. Parents often use it as a reward or a bribe, and children are conditioned from an early age to find comfort in it. If they're allowed to eat sugar, it means they've been 'good'. Sugary bribes are often used to coerce children into doing certain things. When used as a currency, sugar acquires an emotional value: children believe it is special, and they want more of it. You may want to review your parenting style if you've been using sugar as an incentive.

Sugar is known to cause hyperactivity, low concentration and irritability in children. If your children have behavioural problems, progressively decrease the amount of sugar they eat, and replace it with healthier snacks such as fruit kebabs, cheese sticks, peanut or almond butter on rice cakes, sugar-free banana wholemeal muffins, or chips made from leafy greens. Give them only water to drink, starting with diluted fruit juices if they're used to having sodas and soft drinks. Sugar causes tooth decay and gingivitis: another reason to stay away from it, or to be particularly vigilant about tooth hygiene. If you don't help them reduce their sugar intake, your children could suffer weight problems and even eating disorders later on in life.

Sugar may be your security blanket, due to your childhood experiences and the pressure you were under. Sugar may help you deal with stress and dull your emotional pain, while covering up your physical and psychological needs. Only *you* can determine whether you're addicted to sugar to the point of not being able to control your intake. With sugar the problem is the quantity. In small amounts it's certainly not harmful, but in large quantities, it becomes toxic and a poison, just as Dr Lustig suggests.

By using powerful words, Dr Lustig wants to shake us out of our lethargy and wake us up to the fact that sugar is a killer when we consume it excessively. But enjoying the occasional treat is not the same as abusing sugar in a way that causes chronic damage to your body. The decision to quit sugar altogether is up to you. Like an alcoholic who can't stop after the first drink, you might decide that total abstinence is easier than moderation. But if you can control your intake, you don't need such a drastic approach. You can treat yourself daily with small amounts of foods containing sugar or honey. As long as it doesn't lead you to overeat, and as long as your life doesn't depend on it!

When I mention sugar, I don't refer to carbohydrates in general. Sugar is a simple carbohydrate which is quickly absorbed in the bloodstream, causing an unwelcome surge in blood glucose, followed by a 'crash'. Sugar has many names: fructose, maltose, dextrose, lactose, corn syrup, malt syrup, maltodextrin, molasses, honey, maple syrup, fruit juice concentrate, caramel, cane-juice crystals, just to mention a few. Manufacturers often suggest that their products are sugar-free, when in fact they're high in *hidden* simple sugars.

Stick to something natural like an apple or a banana, or make your own healthy, sugar-free cookies. At least you'll know what they contain: sesame oatmeal cookies, banana, chia and oatmeal cookies, carrot or pumpkin oatmeal cookies, oatmeal and pecan cookies. Surf the net for healthy cookie recipes, but consume these treats in moderation.

Slow-release, complex carbohydrates aren't the same as sugar: they are beneficial for weight loss and for your overall health. They help keep your blood sugar level on an even keel. Complex carbohydrates are found in wholegrain breads, whole meal pasta, brown rice, sweet potato, legumes and most vegetables. They give you lasting energy and fill you up.

Currently, there seems to be a war on all carbs, indiscriminately, whether they're simple or complex. Different variations of the Atkins diets with different names are in vogue (the Atkins diet was first launched as 'The Vogue Diet' in an article in Vogue magazine in the early seventies). These high protein, low-carb fad diets have a tendency to put all carbohydrates into the same basket, making them the culprit in obesity. This attitude is misleading and harmful, as it aims at eliminating wholesome foods like beans, potatoes and bananas from your diet. They also advocate excessive amounts of animal protein, which is environmentally unsustainable, and which in the long term can contribute to an array of chronic conditions.

Complex carbs (or high fibre carbs) are an important part of your diet. They give your body a constant supply of fuel, warding off hunger, cravings and energy dips. They are a good source of fibre, which is essential to keep your body healthy. While decreasing your sugar intake, focus on complex carbohydrates to fuel your daily activities and avoid hunger pangs as well as energy dips. Atkins-type high protein diets may show quick results in the short run, but are unsustainable in the long run, as they are too unbalanced and too restrictive. They also lead to fatigue, rebound appetite, slow metabolism and weight gain.

If you want to reduce the amount of sugar you ingest, it may be useful to analyse in what situations you're the most likely to turn to this sweet substance. Maybe you eat sugar to reward yourself. Maybe it nurtures and soothes you, especially in times of anger, sadness, loneliness, insecurity, fear and guilt. Sugar is the fuel that keeps you going, no matter what the feeling is inside.

Sugar enables the brain to produce serotonin, making you feel good. Serotonin is a natural mood-enhancer. But with sugar, the effect is short-lived, and it is wiser to eat complex carbohydrates to obtain a similar, but long-lasting effect. Studies have shown that serotonin is dangerously low in the brains of crash dieters, which makes them feel moody and highly strung. While sugar immediately fixes the problem and will make you instantly feel better, it is not a good medicine, as it leads to further cravings for more sugar.

If you're on a low-calorie, low-carbohydrate diet, your brain may be so depleted of serotonin that sugar feels like a drop of water on a hot stone: the perfect set up for a binge! By including complex carbs in your diet, you won't reach that stage, and you will avoid sweet cravings. Based on hunger, deprivation and serotonin depletion, most ordinary diets don't work in the long run, and will only make you more overweight and depressed, if they don't make you sick.

If you think you're a 'sugarholic', your first step towards recovery is to acknowledge your need for sugar, and the feelings you're trying to repress. When you experience negative emotion such as worry, anxiety or sadness, allow yourself to feel 'the feeling' without attempting to cover it up. Sugar smooths out your problems, but it won't solve them. It will only make them worse, adding more problems to them, such as low self-esteem and powerlessness. The power is yours to stay away from sugar one day at a time.

Key Points and Strategies

- The key with sugar is moderation, not deprivation
- Sugar is addictive and a poison if consumed in excess
- Sugar has many different names and is routinely added to processed foods by manufacturers
- Avoid obvious and hidden sources of sugar, especially in packaged products
- Avoid artificial sweetener
- Drink water instead of soft drinks or diet drinks
- Eat fruit to satisfy your appetite for sugar
- Watch your children's sugar intake
- Don't join the crusade against *all* carbohydrates
- Don't put all carbs into the same basket
- Slow carbs (complex carbs or high fibre carbs) are good for you, as they are absorbed slowly and promote a healthy body
- Slow carbs will help you stick to your diet as they prevent cravings and loss of control
- Sugar, a simple carbohydrate, is absorbed rapidly, resulting in an unnatural blood sugar spike
- Some people may decide to quit sugar altogether to avoid overeating it
- Monitor your emotions and find ways to deal with them without turning to sugar.

18

THE FIBRE MIRACLE

Fibre is a dieter's best friend.

It's not so much what you put into your body that makes you fat; it's what you *don't* put in it! Most Australians don't eat enough fibre. Adults should consume at least 25 - 35 grams of fibre daily, while the average Australian only eats 15 grams.

To reduce your weight, make small, achievable changes to your lifestyle. When you do something over and over, day after day, it becomes automatic. A habit is formed, and it becomes an integral part of you, like the clothes you wear. The more you do something, the less effort it requires.

Drastic changes don't last. They take too much effort, and too much of willpower to be incorporated into your daily routing. To be successful, it's better to take *baby steps*. Although it is advisable to get out of your comfort zone to a certain degree, too much discomfort will take you back to the start. Consider changes that don't frighten you, and that are easy to implement.

A simple and effective way to improve your diet is to add more fibre to it. It will do wonders for your health and kick start your weight loss. By focusing on fibre, you'll make better food choices. Instead of focusing on what you can't eat, put your attention on what you *can* eat: something that will make a big difference to your wellbeing and waistline. Fibre is the secret ingredient to your weight loss success!

Fibre, also known as bulk or roughage, is a carbohydrate that cannot be digested. It is present in all plant foods: fruits, vegetables, grains and legumes. Soluble fibre partially dissolves in water, while insoluble fibre doesn't. This difference is important when it comes to fibre's effect in preventing certain diseases.

- **soluble fibre** includes oatmeal, oat bran, nuts, seeds, legumes, beans, dried peas, lentils, apples, pears, strawberries and blueberries.
- **Insoluble fibre** is found in wholemeal bread, barley, brown rice, bulgur, whole grain breakfast cereals, wheat bran, carrots, cucumber, zucchini, celery and tomatoes.

Fibre can miraculously reduce the risk of developing various conditions, such as high cholesterol, heart disease, diabetes, diverticular disease, haemorrhoids, constipation, colon cancer and possibly even breast cancer. Fibre detoxifies your body, while the larger bulk dilutes carcinogenics and carries them away. When you don't eat enough fibre, toxins that should be eliminated through your bowels get reabsorbed into your bloodstream. Fibre works best in conjunction with water, so make sure you drink enough of it. Eight glasses of water daily is a suggestion, but you may need to drink more depending on the climate you live in, your level of activity and your individual needs.

A recent nurses' health study shows that a diet high in fibre considerably increases life expectancy after a heart attack. This is possibly due to the ability of fibre to soak up excess fat in the bowel, which would normally enter the bloodstream and lead to high cholesterol. High blood cholesterol (LDL = bad cholesterol) leads to *atherosclerosis*. This is a process in which plaque made up of fats and other materials builds up on the walls of your blood vessels, making them stiffer and narrower. Your heart needs to work harder to pump blood into your circulatory system, as the arteries have lost in diameter and elasticity.

High blood pressure contributes to atherosclerosis, by adding extra force against your artery walls, making them more vulnerable to injuries. But high blood pressure is also a direct consequence of the hardening process in your arteries, and in turn leads to more damage. It causes overstretching in weak places, making your blood vessels more prone to rupture, resulting in *strokes* or aneurysms. Vascular scarring occurs due to all the tiny tears that happen over time. These tears and the scar tissue act like nets, catching cholesterol and other debris. Trapped blood may form clots that can further narrow and sometimes block the artery altogether. Eventually, the arteries on the other side of the blockage won't receive enough freshly oxygenated blood, which results in tissue or organ damage. This is what happens during a myocardial infarction (heart attack).

Ten health benefits of a diet high in fibre:

1) Soluble fibre found in beans, oat, flaxseed and oat bran lowers your total blood cholesterol levels by lowering your bad cholesterol
2) Fibre may prevent cancer, by removing poisons and harmful substances that could affect your body cells in a negative way
3) Fibre boosts your immune system, making you less prone to infection and disease, by sweeping the colon

walls, thus preventing pathogens from being reabsorbed via the liver

4) Fibre improves your skin by moving yeast and fungus through the system, rather than allowing them to be excreted through the skin, where they can turn into pimples and rashes

5) Fibre promotes digestive health, preventing constipation, haemorrhoids and diverticular disease (small pouches in your colon). It can also provide relief from irritable bowel syndrome in some people

6) Fibre, in particular soluble fibre, slows the absorption of sugar, stabilizing your blood sugar levels, and thus preventing diabetes. Fibre also plays an important part in the management of type 2 diabetes

7) Fibre helps prevent gallstones by absorbing excess cholesterol in the bowel

8) Fibre-rich foods may prevent the formation of kidney stones

9) Fibre significantly reduces the risk of high blood pressure, heart disease and stroke (if you eat at least 25 g of fibre a day). How much fibre you eat also affects your chances of recovery from a heart attack

10) Fibre is ideal for weight management. It adds bulk without calories to your food, increasing your sense of fullness

Fibre-rich foods require more chewing time, allowing your brain to register when you're no longer hungry, making your less likely to overeat. Fibre-rich foods take longer to eat, and will satisfy you more than foods that are quickly swallowed. If you focus on eating slowly and chewing properly too, your fibre meal will benefit you even more. A meal that is high in complex carbs and fibre will fill you up and keep hunger at bay. Most carbohydrate foods are fibre foods, unless they have been stripped of their natural fibre: this is the case for white flour, white bread, white rice and ordinary pasta. These items are not recommended, or only in extreme cases when nothing else is available. A dish of white pasta with tofu and vegetables for instance can be healthful, when whole meal pasta is not available. Keeping your portions small, the size of a fist or a cup is a safe way to eat, especially at restaurants or parties.

High-fibre foods are often low in calories, especially when compared to foods that are devoid of it. And these calories are not all absorbed by your body, because of the added bulk to your digestive system. As the food transits through your body faster, a percentage of calories remains unutilized and is lost. This is good news if you want to decrease your overall caloric intake. A high-fibre diet increases this helpful wastage of calories.

Fibre acts like a sponge, soaking up water and waste products. Passage through the digestive tract is accelerated and made easier. Waste matters become large and soft and are passed without straining and without putting extra pressure on the wall of the colon. This is why fibre prevents the formation of pouches that are characteristic of diverticulosis. Haemorrhoids are also due to the extra pressure exerted when expelling hard faeces.

A high-fibre diet is the best way to avoid constipation. 'Death begins in the colon' is an old saying and perhaps an oversimplification, but there is some truth in it. General health begins with gastro-intestinal health, and the secret is a diet high in fibre. Avoid refined, processed, low-fibre foods, as well as too much animal fats and protein.

Gut diseases are on the rise and today, they're almost as common as heart disease. They are due to a combination of inadequate diet, lack of exercise and stress. Just by increasing the amount of fibre in every meal you eat, you can start protecting yourself.

Exercise moderately but regularly: For instance, strive for '100 steps per minute' for half an hour a day. Manage your stress with relaxation, meditation and breathing exercises. Don't sweat the small stuff! Live one day at a time, talk to people and adopt the Serenity Prayer as your motto: *God grant me the serenity to accept the things I cannot change, the courage to change the things I can, and the wisdom to know the difference.*

Constipation could contribute to the slow poisoning of the body. And while it may not cause cancer directly, it definitely creates an environment favourable to the development of this disease. Laxatives are not the solution, as they stimulate your bowel artificially to produce a motion. Your bowel becomes *lazy,* and will depend more and more on the effect of laxatives. Laxatives interfere with the internal balance and wisdom of your body. They destroy the natural pattern of bowel movements. Self-induced constipation is the result, which compels you to take more aperients. These may cause diarrhoea and eradicate your bowel flora (good bacteria in your gut), as well as creating mineral imbalances and dehydration. Diarrhoea then leads to even more severe constipation: a vicious circle that you can only break by discontinuing the use of laxatives.

Eat more fresh fruit and vegetables, as well as unrefined carbohydrates like brown rice and whole meal pasta. Barley, oats and oatmeal are also rich in fibre. A slice of whole grain bread has nearly 2g of fibre. You can make your own fibre-rich bread with whole grain flour. Fibre stops you from being hungry, by stabilizing your blood sugar levels, as it encapsulates carbohydrates and makes them less readily available. Energy is released *slowly* into the bloodstream, preventing *hypoglycaemia* (low blood sugar) and cravings. Fibre also prevents your brain from being depleted of serotonin, especially when you eat a combination of fibre and complex carbohydrates.

While type 1 diabetes is mainly due to genetic factors, type 2 diabetes is often linked to obesity and metabolic syndrome. A lack of fibre contributes to the development of this condition, as well as an over-consumption of refined sugar and high fructose corn syrup in processed foods and soft drinks (sodas). This puts undue strain on your insulin system, making it inefficient after some time. The insulin response is triggered by sugar in your blood. If there is too much sugar, there will be too much insulin. The result is rebound hypoglycaemia, and this yo-yo effect may eventually cause a fault in your body's ability to produce and utilize insulin.

A diabetic's blood sugar rises too high, and there is no, or insufficient, insulin, or the cells fail to respond to the normal actions of the hormone. The body still produces insulin, but the cells in the body become resistant to it and are unable to use it as effectively, leading to *hyperglycaemia* (high blood sugar).

Fibre helps prevent diabetes, as it delays the digestion of carbohydrates. Complex carbohydrates, naturally rich in fibre, are absorbed slowly. Their energy reaches the bloodstream progressively, while insulin is released at the same slow and steady rate, preventing spikes and drops in blood sugar levels.

Increase the amount of fibre you ingest gradually, to allow your body to get used to it. There may be an adjustment phase, especially if you haven't touched a vegetable since you were six years old! *Flatulence* could be an unwelcome side effect, but you will overcome it as you persist in eating a diet high in fibre. Probiotics can reduce flatulence. They are beneficial bacteria found in natural, unsweetened yoghourt, as well as in probiotic supplements available from health stores and chemists. Useful in fighting off harmful bacteria, they will boost your overall wellbeing and immune function. These micro-organisms assist the digestive process in the gut.

If you keep experiencing digestive discomfort, increase the number of small meals you have. Several small meals are easier to digest than three big ones, and breaking up your calories will stimulate your metabolism. If you're very sensitive to the effect of fibre, try not eating more than one 'gassy' item per meal. For instance, don't combine broccoli with beans and wholemeal pasta.

Tips to increase the amount of fibre in your diet:

- Sprinkle oat or wheat bran on your porridge, breakfast cereals, soups, sauces and salads
- Always use whole grain products
- Use super foods like chia and quinoa
- Eat plenty of vegetables and have fresh fruit for dessert or a snack
- Gradually increase your consumption of beans, peas, chick peas and other legumes
- Include seeds and nuts in your daily diet
- Switch to wholemeal pasta and brown rice
- Add flaxseed to yoghurt, smoothies or onto cooked vegetables
- Try tofu and tempeh instead of meat
- Experiment with vegetarian curries and casseroles
- Go berserk with homemade soups and salads!

Make a slimming 'fibre soup' by combining these ingredients in a big pan with filtered water:

- Onion, ginger and garlic (pre-fried in a little coconut oil)
- Carrots and celery
- Capsicum (bell peppers): red, green and yellow
- Pumpkin or sweet potato
- Potato
- Creamed corn

- A teaspoon of tomato paste
- Curry, nutmeg or herbs and spices according to taste.

Toss up these ingredients for a fresh summer salad:

- Onion
- Lettuce
- Baby spinach
- Tomatoes
- Cucumber
- Capsicums
- Balsamic vinegar or lemon juice
- Extra virgin olive oil
- Garlic and fresh herbs to taste.

Mix these ingredients for a convenient and nutritious bean salad, full of fibre, complex carbohydrates and vegetable protein:

- Baked beans (drained of excess sauce)
- Three or four bean mix (drained and rinsed)
- Corn kernels
- Frozen peas (defrosted)
- Chopped onion, spring onion or chives
- Garlic (optional)
- Chopped parsley, basil, tarragon or coriander
- Vinegar of lemon juice.

BROCCOLI is 'miracle' vegetable containing iron, calcium, magnesium, folic acid, vitamin A and C. It is also thought to have anti-cancer properties. Eat broccoli at least two or three times a week, raw in salads or lightly cooked in stir-fries. Add it to soups, curries and casseroles.

For an easy and delicious stir-fry, chop and combine the following ingredients in a wok or big pan, using organic coconut oil (best cooking oil as it is not altered by heat):

- Onion, ginger and garlic
- Broccoli
- Red, green and yellow capsicums
- Carrots (in fine stripes)
- Cabbage
- Fresh mushrooms
- Low sodium soy sauce and/or satay sauce
- Add strips of lean beef, chicken breast or diced firm tofu for protein.

Preparation is essential for effective weight loss, and it's easy with a few basic recipes and a little organization. These dishes can be prepared in advance. Enjoy them with brown rice, quinoa, whole meal pasta, or simply with a slice of whole grain bread. The vegetable soup and bean salad are filling and guaranteed not to leave you hungry. You can take them to work for a healthy lunch. Always carry fruit with you such as apples, pears or bananas in case you need a snack. Dried fruit and nuts are handy when you're craving sweet foods. Develop an interest in healthy cooking and start collecting your favourite recipes. Draw up a meal plan for the week ahead and put all the ingredients you need on your shopping list.

You can rely on fibre-rich foods to supply you with lasting fuel, as well as an array of valuable nutrients, essential vitamins, minerals and trace elements. Focus on fibre, as it fills you up and makes you slim. Fibre foods are your best friends when embarking on a weight loss journey!

Key Points and Strategies:

- Focus on what you can have (= fibre-rich foods), rather than what you can't have
- Remember that only plant foods contain fibre
- Fibre prevents constipation, heart disease, type 2 diabetes and cancer
- Fibre detoxifies your body
- Fibre is perfect for weight loss, as it saves calories and prevents hunger attacks
- Eat plenty of fruit, vegetables, legumes, brown rice, whole meal pasta and whole grain bread
- Add oat bran, chia, flaxseed, seeds and nuts to your diet
- Gradually increase the amount of fibre you eat, to allow your digestive system to adjust to it
- Avoid eating several 'gassy' items at the same time
- Use probiotics (yoghourt or supplements) if excessive flatulence occurs

19

SHAKE THE SALT HABIT

Reducing your salt intake is part of a healthy diet. Too much salt can lead to high blood pressure, stroke, heart disease and kidney failure.

NaCl, a chemical compound made of sodium and chloride is not a spice but a *mineral.* Salt is the only rock we eat. While salt is probably the most popular and well-known flavour enhancer, it can be *harmful,* as opposed to spices. Spices come from living organisms, provide aroma and taste to cooking. Besides, they have many healthful benefits and are generally used more sparsely than salt.

Salt has been important to humans for thousands of years, not primarily for its taste, but for its ability to preserve food, especially meat and fish. This was one of the foundations of civilization. People didn't have to depend on seasonal availability of food, and it allowed them to travel over long distances. Salt was difficult to obtain and very pricey, which made it a highly valued trade item. In some places, it was even considered a currency.

Roman soldiers were paid in salt, which is the origin of the word *salary*. Many salt roads, such as the Via Salaria (an ancient Roman road in Italy), had been established since the Bronze Age, which began in the third millennium BC. Today salt is cheap and ubiquitous: it is used in cooking, and it is present in most processed items, including sweet foods such as biscuits, cakes and chocolates. *Saltiness* is one of the basic human tastes, besides sweet, bitter and sour.

Salt is essential for life as the body can't produce it on its own. It is necessary for maintaining adequate blood pressure, by keeping water in your blood vessels. This mineral allows you to retain enough fluid to hydrate your body. If you ingest too much salt, you will retain too much fluid, which may cause health problems like high blood pressure and oedema (swelling).

The Heart Foundation sets the maximum limit for sodium intake at 2300 mg a day (less for children), which is the equivalent of one teaspoon of salt. People with high blood pressure or diabetes are told not to exceed 1500 mg of sodium a day. While the World Health Organization advises consumers not to go over 5000 mg a day, many people consume twice as much and more!

Your total sodium intake doesn't just include table salt, but all salts: rock salt, sea salt, salt flakes, pink salt, garlic salt, onion salt, seasoning, monosodium glutamate (MSG), stock cubes, soy sauce and other ready-to-use sauces. It includes *hidden* salt in supermarket products like frozen meals, canned vegetables, popular cereals, cheeses, processed meats and potato chips (crisps). Because of these non-obvious sources of salt, your salt intake may be high without you being aware of it – another good reason to avoid processed, packaged foods and takeaways (the same items that are also high in trans fat and sugar). Like most people who've been eating mindlessly, you may need to cut down your salt intake.

Many foods contain small amounts of sodium naturally, and theoretically you don't need to add extra salt to your meals, unless you're in a hot environment or do a lot of strenuous exercise. In this case, you will need to increase your water intake simultaneously. Sodium binds water in your bloodstream, and while dehydration can occur if you don't drink enough, it can also happen if you don't get enough salt. Too little salt can be just as harmful as too much. Celery, carrots, spinach and beetroot are naturally high in sodium, but they're good for you too: these are vegetables you should eat when you've been sweating a lot.

There are at least ten conditions that are caused or worsened by excess dietary salt:

1) Hypertension (=high blood pressure) can generally be defined as a blood pressure of 140/90 mmHg or over. High blood pressure is the biggest cause of death in the world, due to the strokes and heart attacks it contributes to. A diet high in salt and low in potassium disrupts the natural sodium-potassium balance in the body. This leads to fluid retention, which increases the pressure exerted by the blood against the blood vessel walls.

Your body is designed for a high-potassium diet, not a high-salt diet. It is estimated that a reduction in salt intake from 10 g a day to 6 g would reduce blood pressure to the extent that it could reduce mortality from strokes by 16% and mortality from coronary heart disease by 12%. Other factors contributing to hypertension are: low consumption of fruit and vegetables (low potassium intake), obesity, excess alcohol and lack of physical exercise. Diabetes also leads to high blood pressure and heart problems, as it damages arteries, making them harder (=atherosclerosis).

2) Osteoporosis is a condition involving the thinning of the bones, which are depleted of calcium, thus becoming brittle and more prone to fractures. A high salt intake leaches calcium from the bones, while increasing calcium losses in the urine. Over an extended period, this leads to weakening of the bones and osteoporosis. Reducing your salt intake is more effective than taking a calcium supplement to prevent this condition. Lack of exercise, lack of vitamin D, magnesium deficiency, smoking and heavy drinking are also risk factors for osteoporosis.

3) Kidney disease. Your blood is filtered through your kidneys, via osmosis, to draw excess water out of your blood. This requires a balance of sodium and potassium. A diet high in salt alters this balance, leading to reduced kidney function. Your kidneys remove less fluid from your body, which results in high blood pressure. This puts extra strain on your kidneys and could lead to a deterioration of their function.

4) Kidney stones. Urinary calcium, the main constituent of kidney stones, is increased by a diet high in salt. This increases the risk of stones forming. A number of studies have conclusively shown that a reduction in dietary salt reduces calcium excretion, therefore reducing the incidence of renal stones. People with high blood pressure are also more likely to develop kidney stones: another reason to eat less salt.

5) Fatty liver disease is the build-up of excess fat in the liver cells. It affects about one in ten people in Australia. It is normal for the liver to contain some fat, but if it accounts for over a tenth of the liver's weight, you have fatty liver and this could cause serious complications. Your liver can become inflamed, which could lead to scarring, cirrhosis and ultimately liver failure.

Salt contributes to this condition because it increases your blood pressure and makes your kidneys work harder. When the kidneys are overworked, the liver picks up the pieces, taking over some of the kidneys' functions. This leads to the liver being overworked and possibly damaged. High-salt processed foods such as manufactured meats, bacon and sausages are probably the worst culprits as they're also high in nitrates, nitrites, colourings, flavourings, sweeteners and trans fats. The main causes of fatty liver disease are excess weight, obesity, diabetes and chronic alcohol abuse.

6) Increased risk of stomach cancer, especially if you eat more than 6 g of salt a day. Stomach cancer is the fourth most common cancer in the world (in men the top three cancers are lung, prostate and bowel; in women they are breast, bowel and cervix). Several studies have evidenced the relationship between salt or salted foods and increased stomach cancer risk. The average salt intake in each population is closely related to gastric cancer mortality. In Japan for instance there are four times as many cases as in the United Kingdom, possibly due to the high salt content of the traditional Japanese diet.

7) Salt exacerbates chronic asthma. A diet high in salt has been proven to make asthma worse, by reducing the total amount of air expired. A diet *low* in salt produces less *inflammation,* which is beneficial as people need to use their bronchodilator drug less often.

8) Dehydration. The more salt you eat, the more water you need to drink in order for your body to dilute the excess salt. If you fail to increase your water intake according to your salt consumption, you will become *dehydrated.* Salt makes you thirsty, but by the time you feel thirst, the dehydration process is already under way. Signs of dehydration are fatigue, irritability and brain fog, as well as little or no urine. Any urine that is produced is *darker* than normal.

9) Headaches. The majority of headaches are caused by a *potassium* deficiency, which in turn is caused by excess sodium. Potassium is primarily contained in your body cells, whereas sodium is contained in your bloodstream. Both these minerals attract water ions, competing for water. When your diet is too high in sodium, your blood holds more sodium ions, and therefore more water is attracted into your bloodstream. This same water leaves your body cells, causing them to become dehydrated. When the cells in your brain become dehydrated, you have a headache. You can take painkillers, but this won't address the cause of the problem. Your cells need more water, which has been taken away from them due to the sodium overload in your bloodstream.

10) Weight gain due to water retention. While salt alone doesn't cause your body to gain or lose fat, as it has no calories, it leads to bloating and puffiness, a 'waterlogged' feeling. If you eat too much salt, your weight will fluctuate, as your body will hold on to more water in order to compensate for the salt in your bloodstream. Once you cut down on salt and drink enough water, you will see the swelling diminish, and your weight might drop considerably. Add fresh *lemon* or lime juice to your water, because lemons are diuretic. Lemons assist kidney and liver function. Outside the body, lemon juice is acidic, but inside the body it promotes an alkaline environment. Once it has been fully metabolized and its minerals are dissociated in the bloodstream, lemon juice has an alkalizing effect and raises the pH of your body (pH above 7 is alkaline).

Salt is naturally present at low levels in all foods, but around 80 % of our salt intake is hidden in processed foods. Your health is your wealth, and your choices today will determine your wellbeing tomorrow. A completely salt-free diet is theoretically impossible and not necessary, as some salt is beneficial and prevents you from getting dehydrated. But you don't need the massive amounts of salt that are present in takeaway and manufactured foods.

Focus on fresh products like fruit and vegetables. Look for 'no added salt' labels in your supermarket. Get rid of your salt shaker, or hide it for the occasional visitor who may ask for it. Perhaps you believe that salt makes food tasty, but it actually masks the real taste of food. At first, you will find that everything tastes bad without salt, but you will soon realize that salt is only a habit, an acquired taste.

Once you get used to a diet low in sodium, you will want to continue eating that way, as it is more satisfying, and you will begin to feel better. You will begin tasting your food properly, maybe for the first time in your life. You will probably feel less thirsty and maybe you will need to drink less. This is natural, as the water you drink helps dilute excess salt in your bloodstream, and decrease bloating: the more salt you eat, the more water you need to drink.

With salt all foods taste the same: *salty*. Experiment with herbs and spices instead. They enhance flavour and also have healing properties. Your taste buds will recover and, after a while, you will begin to enjoy the real taste of food. Salt will seem uniforming, boring and even unpleasant in comparison. Without added salt, your food will taste more delicious than ever!

Key Points and Strategies:

- Salt is necessary for survival, but most people ingest too much of it
- All foods naturally contain salt, so you don't need to add it to your food
- Become aware of the food choices you make
- Most of the salt you get is hidden in takeaway and processed foods
- Excessive salt is linked to high blood pressure and heart diseases
- Excessive salt leads to osteoporosis, liver and kidney problems (including kidney stones)

- Salt can cause you to retain excess water, adding to your weight
- Focus on fresh products like fruit and vegetables instead of manufactured items
- Throw the salt out of the shaker; fill it with other tasty mixtures: herbs, spices or sesame seeds.

20

ALCOHOL AND WEIGHT LOSS DO NOT GO TOGETHER

Most people who consume alcohol don't have a drinking problem. However, alcohol can be a problem when you intend to lose weight or maintain your current shape. This is due to at least six different reasons:

1) Alcoholic drinks are high in calories

They are made by fermenting and distilling natural starch and sugar. Alcohol contains seven calories per gram, almost as many as pure fat. A glass of wine can have the same calories as four cookies, and a pint of lager (about half a litre) has the calorific equivalent of a slice of pizza. Calories from alcohol are 'empty': they have no nutritional value. Alcoholic drinks may contain traces of vitamins and minerals, but not in amounts capable of making any significant contribution to your diet.

2) Alcohol makes you hungry

By stimulating the *hypothalamus,* a part of the brain that regulates things like body temperature, circadian rhythms, and most importantly HUNGER, alcohol makes you feel hungry at a time when you wouldn't normally desire food

By promoting extra *insulin* release from your pancreas, which causes a drop in blood sugar (hypoglycaemia), alcohol creates a sudden and strong craving for sugary and starchy foods.

3) Alcohol makes you crave fatty and salty foods

Fatty foods soothe your stomach, as alcohol causes inflammation of the stomach lining. Salt alleviates the *dehydration* caused by alcohol. Alcohol acts on the kidneys, and it makes you pass more urine than you can take in. A powerful diuretic, it extracts fluids from your body and leads to dehydration, which causes the nausea, headache and dry mouth associated with hangovers.

4) Alcohol boosts your appetite and triggers unhealthy longings for junk food. This may be due to alcohol's effect on the main inhibitory transmitter in the brain: GABA. When you consume alcohol, it attaches itself to this neurotransmitter, slowing things down and reducing stress and anxiety levels. Your self-control diminishes, and you feel less guilty than usual about devouring a greasy slice of pizza or some fried chicken and fries. The health-conscious part of your brain tends to be switched off when you drink!

5) Alcohol slows your metabolism. While your liver is busy processing alcohol, it puts calorie burning on the back burner. The liver's priority is to rid the body of alcohol's by-products, which it recognizes as *toxins*. While you can store protein, carbohydrates and fat in your body, you can't store alcohol. Your system wants to eliminate it as soon as possible, so other tasks like absorbing nutrients and burning fat are interrupted.

6) Alcohol affects the body's endocrine system (your hormones). High alcohol consumption leads to high *cortisol* levels. Cortisol is a stress hormone, and its release over an extended period of time causes health problems: fatigue, hypertension, ulcers, cancer, premature aging, depression, impaired immune system, blood sugar abnormalities, and... weight gain, in particular around the abdomen (pot belly). Belly fat is the worst kind of fat, as it increases the likelihood of high cholesterol, high blood pressure, insulin resistance, diabetes and cardiovascular disease. Visceral fat cells produce hormones that regulate weight and appetite, which can lead to further weight gain and increased feelings of hunger.

While excessive alcohol consumption is harmful, especially for your liver, moderate drinking can offer some benefits. Alcohol has been proven to lower your risk of cardiovascular disease, due to its *blood thinning* properties and possibly due to its *relaxing* effect. Alcohol can help you unwind after a hectic day and reduce stress. Tasty and enjoyable, it complements a nice meal, and it is there to celebrate special occasions like weddings and parties.

As a mood enhancer, it can add something to your life experience. It can be a way to open up and make new friends for someone with mild social anxiety, even though there is a risk of becoming dependent if you use it for this purpose. Alcohol produces *euphoria,* which is only temporary though. Once the relaxing effect is over, you may feel worse, as your serotonin levels plummet as soon as alcohol leaves your body. This serotonin depletion can easily lead to cravings and food binges.

Every time you drink, you reinforce the 'good feeling', and you could end up relying on it. Alcohol is a calmative and it blots out unwanted feelings you may find painful or disturbing. But problems don't go away just because you momentarily escape from them. In social situations, alcohol can mask shyness, but it doesn't solve the emotional conflict that is at the origin of shyness and low self-esteem.

If you choose to drink, limit yourself to one small glass a day, preferably with a meal. Follow these principles if you wish to drink sensibly, especially in social situations:

- Know your limit and plan in advance how much you will drink
- Delay your first drink for as long as possible
- Accept a drink only when you really want one
- If you don't want it, decline with a polite 'No, thank you', and no details
- Choose quality rather than quantity
- Choose a low alcohol drink like a light beer
- Eat food while your drink and never drink on an empty stomach
- Slowly sip your drink
- Don't drain your glass, as it may be a cue to your host that you would like a refill
- Keep track of how much you drink
- Alternate alcoholic drinks with non-alcoholic drinks like water or diluted fruit juices.

Alcohol can increase HDL, the 'good' cholesterol, if used *moderately* and in the context of a healthy diet, along with regular physical activity. Higher HDL levels are linked to lower risks of cardiovascular disease. Red wine is beneficial in small amounts, as it contains a naturally-occurring, powerful *polyphenol* that has significant antioxidant properties. This plant-derived compound is found in the skin and seeds of grapes. Since red wines have extended contact time with the grape's skin during fermentation, they will have higher levels of *resveratrol.*

In any case, cutting down on drinking will have a positive effect on weight loss and maintaining a healthy weight.

Key Points and Strategies:

- Alcohol is fattening and not recommended as part of a weight loss program
- Alcohol is a mood-altering substance and regular consumption could lead to dependence
- Moderate amounts of red wine can be good for your heart
- Stick to one small glass a day if you wish to drink
- Use specific techniques to drink less in social situations.

21

. . . .

ARE YOU A DIET PERFECTIONIST?

. . . .

Perfectionism is self-abuse and creates the perfect conditions for self-sabotage.

You may encounter many hurdles, but more than anything else, perfectionism is likely to ruin your diet. It is a prescription for failure, and a precursor to eating disorders. If diet after diet is a disaster for you, it's time to adopt a flexible approach to losing weight and maintaining your new shape, one that is comfortable and works for you over a long period of time, preferably for the rest of your life. You don't need to diet perfectly and follow a plan to the letter to achieve your goal. The 'all or nothing' attitude is unrealistic, as it is natural for humans to make mistakes.

Some behaviour patterns can sabotage your weight loss efforts:

- Intending to start your diet *tomorrow* or on a Monday
- Using the words 'good' and 'bad' to describe foods and your eating behaviour

- Wanting to accelerate the process by eating less than your diet prescribes
- Feeling hungry and deprived all the time
- Exercising too often and too strenuously
- Eliminating all your favourite treats
- Giving up as soon as you 'fall off the wagon'
- Thinking that *one* mistake has ruined your diet and punishing yourself for it
- Thinking that your failure is due to your lack of effort and perseverance.

Some suggestions to keep on top of a healthy eating plan:

- Acknowledge that you won't change overnight: it takes time to form new habits and to incorporate them into your daily life
- Stick to a regular meal pattern, e.g. three main meals and three snacks, to ward off hunger pangs and keep temptation at bay
- Drink more water: one glass *before* each meal, and one more *with* each meal. Drink a glass of water in every meeting or conference call at work. Drink a glass of water first thing in the morning and last thing in the evening, after completing all your tasks. These small changes can quickly add up to the desirable eight glasses a day
- Keep a food diary: write down everything you eat and drink. Research shows that this is an effective way to increase your weight loss
- Cement a moderate exercise program into your daily routine. A half-hour walk can make a huge difference, but don't beat yourself up if you skip it once in a while
- Don't eliminate everything from your diet at once. Cut things down progressively, one item at a time. For instance, you could start by drinking your tea or coffee

without sugar. Give yourself plenty of time to adjust to changes. The same applies to portions: reduce them gradually

- Allow for a high-calorie treat now and again, preferably something small
- Don't confine yourself to a strict diet plan with no end in sight, as you will quickly feel overwhelmed and discouraged
- Don't feel guilty if you slip up or fail to exercise on the odd occasion.

To endure starvation and deprivation may be useful for a short period of time, but it will backfire in the long run. Crash diets are the cause of rebound hunger, bingeing and renewed weight gain: the yo-yo effect. The 'all or nothing' attitude doesn't work. A more sensible approach is to admit that you're not perfect. To avoid disappointment, don't expect too much of yourself. If you believe you can stick to a restricted plan all the time, you're kidding yourself. If you believe you can control yourself around food all the time, especially when eating out, you'll punish yourself as soon as you make a mistake.

You've been following a strict eating plan for a while but suddenly, you can't help it and reach out for that dreaded piece of cake. You loathe yourself for being so weak, as you expected yourself to be *perfect* all the time. You're disappointed and decide to give up your diet, at least until the next day. You decide to stuff yourself with food. The next day, you punish yourself by starving yourself and enduring a gruelling workout session at the gym. This is the cycle of guilt and punishment that inevitably leads to binging and deprivation.

People who succeed in losing weight the healthy way are those who don't have unrealistic expectations of themselves. They know what they want, while being aware that they can't be perfect.

They have a more relaxed approach to weight loss and weight maintenance. They routinely allow themselves to have 'bad' foods like chocolate *without* feeling bad about it.

Being flexible and admitting that you can't be strong all the time is your foundation for success. Temptation is everywhere, and the more you deprive yourself, the more you're likely to give in to your desires. But willpower is also a muscle that you can train and gets stronger with regular use.

Willpower is energy, and, to avoid using it up too quickly, give in to your desires from time to time, in a controlled way. Allow yourself a favourite food at least once or twice a week. Prescribe it to yourself as a preventative, and make it an integral part of your diet. Consciously choosing to have a treat will stop you from feeling guilty. You won't be disappointed in yourself, as your indulgence will be included in your plan. You won't need to punish yourself for stepping out of line. Giving in to temptation is not the end of the world, and certainly not the end of your diet. Enjoy your treat as much as possible, every bite of it! Then immediately go back to your healthy eating program.

You don't have to be perfect, and you don't have to be good all the time. Eat sensibly today, without regretting what happened yesterday, and without worrying about what might happen tomorrow. Congratulate yourself for doing well *today*. If you overeat, it's not a catastrophe. You can correct and overcome your mistakes. If you've gorged on a tub of ice cream, don't scold yourself or put yourself down. Don't think you should abandon your diet just because you overate.

Apply these strategies when you feel your resolve weakening:

1. Remind yourself that it's okay to stray occasionally. You can take control of the situation and go back to where you were.

Overcoming challenges will add to your experience, as well as making you stronger and more confident

2. Go for a 30 minute walk. Exercise will clear your mind, oxygenate your lungs, boost your metabolism and help your body burn the excess energy you've consumed. You can also do some Pilates or yoga stretches

3. Stock your fridge with carrots, apples, celery sticks or other crunchy vegetables. You can chew on them when you're feeling stressed (sugar-free chewing gum may also help). Stress is the quickest way to deplete your willpower, so it's important to give yourself a *break*. Do what you can to eliminate stress from your life, or learn how to handle it in a constructive manner.

4. Prevention is better than a cure when it comes to cravings. Eat fibre and complex carbohydrates to fill you up and satisfy your hunger and appetite. Eat frequently, whenever you feel hungry. Regular eating, in the form of six small, nutritious meals a day, is the secret to successful dieting.

5. Take time to play and enjoy yourself. Create a balance between work and pleasure in your life. Recreation is important to 're-create' yourself. Losing weight can be hard work, and it can be frustrating. You need to look after yourself or you will start resenting your diet. A new project, a movie, a book, your favourite TV series, or simply a few minutes on your own, breathing deeply, can help lift your mood and recharge your batteries. Friendship and love are essential in a world that sometimes seems uncaring.

6. Repetition is the key to adopting new habits. If you practice the principles outlined in this book, they will become part of your routine, a new way of life. Little by little, you can incorporate healthy changes into your lifestyle, but you don't have to live like that all the time. Eating what you want without guilt is better than constantly feeling deprived and frustrated. Overly strict eating plans don't work, as they take away your freedom: you feel incarcerated. As a result you rebel and binge on 'bad' foods. Excess weight could be a sign that there is too much *control* in your life. But if you know that you're allowed to eat what you want, any time you want, you won't feel the urge to rebel and splurge on forbidden foods. The knowledge that you have a choice helps you break free from compulsive eating, as compulsive behaviour can only exist if there is no choice.

7. Feeling good is your number one priority. A diet shouldn't be torture or punishment. Instead, it's an opportunity to improve your health as well as your self-esteem. If you fail today, don't blame yourself and don't dwell on it. Just start again the next day. Every day is a new beginning.

Everyone gets tempted, and food is especially tempting: it's always there, and it looks and smells so delicious. You need to eat every day, and you can't just give up eating like someone would give up smoking or drinking. To give in to temptation allows you to feel free. The biggest temptation is to ditch your diet, and overcoming it will make you grow as an individual. It's the power of endurance: an opportunity to renew your commitment, strengthen your determination and pave your way for success.

Key Points and Strategies:

- Avoid perfectionism and the 'all or nothing' mindset
- Wanting to be perfect all the time is guaranteed to make you fail
- Adopt a flexible attitude and be lenient towards yourself
- Don't force yourself to adhere to a rigid eating plan
- Don't restrict calories or certain foods too much
- Eat regularly and drink plenty of water
- Exercise moderately to increase your wellbeing

- Make frequent treats an integral part of your diet
- Don't quit your diet if you slip up, as it is normal to make mistakes
- *Learn* from your mistakes instead of criticizing and punishing yourself
- It takes time to form new habits. Implement changes progressively
- Willpower is a limited resource, so don't expect too much of yourself
- Avoid stress and learn how to cope with it
- Take time to enjoy and re-create yourself, in order to recharge your batteries
- Be aware that you are a *free* individual and that you have choices
- Make *feeling good* your number one priority!

22

PREPARE YOURSELF

Successful weight loss starts in the mind.

Before you decide to go on a weight loss journey, prepare yourself mentally: do some 'brain surgery' and cut out beliefs that are unrealistic and counterproductive. Replace them with ideas that will work for you.

Cross out the idea that you can lose a big amount of weight quickly: it's impossible and unhealthy, as well as unsustainable in the long run. If you set yourself unrealistic expectations, you will regain any weight lost as soon as you go off your diet.

Another mistake is to believe that all you need is to lose the kilograms that you've set out to lose, and you'll be done. Nothing is further from the truth. Losing weight is not your biggest job. After reaching a healthy weight, your main objective is to maintain it for the rest of your life, while enjoying a lifestyle that will promote your wellbeing at all levels.

Ask yourself if this is the right time for you to lose weight. Don't do it in the middle of a crisis– a financial struggle, job change, moving houses, separation or divorce or the loss of a loved one. If you have to take exams in the near future, focus on your studies, rather than your waist line. Prioritize. Weight loss comes *after,* when you'll have more time to exercise and design meal plans. Eat well during exams, but if you don't have time to cook proper meals, take a vitamin and mineral supplement. You'll also benefit from taking a Ginkgo Biloba supplement to enhance your memory and concentration, as this herb increases blood flow to the brain.

Think about how to make your weight loss journey easier:

Read this book and keep it handy. Refer to the Strategies at the end of each chapter as often as possible, to imprint them in your mind. Also read *The Magic of Willpower:* it will help you along the way, especially if you have trouble staying motivated and sticking with your new resolutions

Consult a *dietician,* particularly if you have special needs, like diabetes or food allergies. A dietician will create meal plans tailored to your requirements, and suited to your lifestyle, taste, preferences and conditions

Your *doctor* can give you a physical examination and rule out conditions that could affect your metabolism, like a hormone imbalance or an underactive thyroid. Other factors that could slow your metabolism are old age (there is no cure for that), stress, worries, lack of sleep, certain medications, a diet high in saturated fats and trans fats, and a lack of exercise in general

Hire a *personal trainer,* or enrol in a *yoga* or *Pilates* class. Join a *walking* or *hiking* group or club. If you can't find one in your area, start your own! Suggest it to your friends, neighbours, colleagues, or parents and teachers at your children's school. It's a great way to socialize and lift depression.

Find out as much as possible about healthy eating. This kind of research will prepare you mentally. Surf the net for tips and recipes, but stay away from methods that promise a quick fix. Fad diets and miracle cures don't work, but you can be tempted to fall for them. Don't waste your time, money and efforts. The only way to lose weight effectively and permanently is to do it slowly and gradually. If a diet guarantees a rapid weight reduction, it means you'll regain your kilograms rapidly too.

Guilt is the main roadblock to putting yourself first, but the more you do for yourself, the less likely you will be to overeat. While you can still give to others, acknowledge the importance of your *own* needs, like sleep, relaxation and recreation. This is a healthy way to be 'selfish': you will be a better person and better able to look after others if you're well-rested and in a good mood.

Mothers have a tendency to put others before themselves, especially if they care for young children. No matter what you circumstances are, don't neglect to make time for yourself: it will help you be a more balanced person. Your family will not miss out; they will benefit from it. If people ask too much of you, don't be afraid to be assertive and to say no. Your wellbeing is more important than being at everyone's beck and call. Learn to work smarter and master the art of delegation.

You don't have to be perfect, and you don't have to stick to a strict diet plan. This way, you can free yourself of the destructive cycle of *guilt* and *punishment*. You are the only one who decides *what* you eat, *when* and *how much*. The occasional indulgence won't harm you and can even be good for you, as it will keep you on the right track without depleting your willpower.

Accept your body as it is *now*, even though you may be obese or overweight. How can you like yourself now, when you're so fat? If you start loving yourself now, and start loving your body, you will make your journey a pleasant one, and you will cultivate a mindset for permanent weight loss. Hating your current shape won't make it disappear. You can't lose fat by loathing it. Dissatisfaction with your body leads to crash diets, and failure with these diets is only too predictable: your self-esteem plummets, and your weight rises. If you love your body despite its imperfections, your self-esteem will increase, and your weight will drop. Make a decision to accept your body instead of fighting against it.

Losing weight and keeping it off is a lifelong task. Prepare yourself to change your eating habits and embrace a new way of life. This is *your* journey. As you become aware of the food you eat and the exercise you do, you will begin to enjoy these changes while they gradually become a part of you.

Concentrate on being healthy rather than losing weight. See your journey as something exciting and enjoyable that you're doing for yourself and that you're looking forward to. This will enable you to shift your focus and look at it from a positive angle. You will be able to let go of your fat without having to struggle. You will be so busy enjoying your new lifestyle that you won't have time to worry about excess kilograms. You will lose weight naturally, thanks to your new outlook and the new habits you've acquired.

Key Points and Strategies:

- Good preparation is essential for success – and it always begins in the mind
- Choose your timing and avoid dieting during periods of stress and crisis
- Use all the tools available, including this book

- See your doctor for a physical examination and to eliminate certain conditions
- Hire a dietician or a personal trainer if necessary
- Learn as much as possible about healthy eating and living
- Look after yourself body and mind: learn to put yourself first
- Make a conscious decision *not* to be a diet perfectionist
- Love your body *now*, even though you may be overweight or obese
- Your diet is in *your* hands: *you* choose what you will eat, when and how much
- Be prepared to adopt lifelong eating and lifestyle habits
- Be prepared to lose weight slowly and gradually.

23

EMOTIONAL ROADBLOCKS

When you're overweight or obese, your self-esteem drops. You suffer. You're scared people might judge you and find you unattractive.

Why would anyone want to be overweight, when it is connected with so much emotional pain, judgment of others and self-condemnation? It is generally accepted that people are overweight because they eat too much and they don't exercise enough. But why would they allow themselves to get that way in the first place? There is a combination of motives that compels a person to put on excessive weight. These motives are complex and mostly *subconscious*. It will be up to you to bring to light your own reasons and unravel them, using introspection and insight, with the help of counselling or psychotherapy if necessary.

Sometimes overwhelming things happen in your life, and you lose track of your weight while busy dealing with something else. This happens with parenthood, for instance. A new baby is such a big change that everything else goes on the back burner. Health challenges also influence your shape, and some conditions can trigger weight gain, such as hypothyroidism or depression. Sadly, a lot of people were abused as children, physically, emotionally or sexually, which can lead to being overweight or obese later on in life.

You can never judge a person without knowing their full story. It may be possible that fat contributes to a sense of strength and stability when everything else is crumbling and appears flimsy. Fat can be a protective armour against emotional distress. Perhaps you have a deeply engrained fear of living, of taking risks and being hurt or disappointed. Bad experiences have made you *insecure* and reticent.

Heavy people seem strong on the outside, because they have more force than lighter people. In Sumo wrestling, massive men tend to do best, using their imposing girth to gain necessary leverage. But heavy people could also be stronger on the inside. Fat insulates them against what they fear the most: their *own* feelings. It cushions them from the blows dished out by a world is perceived as hostile.

As children, you noticed that grownups were so much bigger than yourself. You respected and perhaps feared them for that reason, while feeling protected by their strong presence. As an adult, you tend to react similarly to someone with a large body. At a subconscious level, overweight people might be aware that their size gives them more presence and substance. They seem to possess more power and authority. They come across as more resilient and reliable, not only physically, but also mentally.

When you're overweight, you may feel strong and inspire trust and deference. At the same time, you may fear what people say behind your back. A lot of people in leading positions are overweight, but that could be due to the long hours they spend sitting in front of a computer screen. *Stress* and being overworked are also contributing factors.

Subconsciously, you may believe that the heavier you are, the less likely you are to be pushed around and manipulated by others. In reality this doesn't quite work though, and overweight people are often discriminated against, whether for job applications or to get the medical care they need. According to British research, heavy patients are less likely to be treated with respect, and more likely to be the butt of jokes. They are often banned from routine surgery, including knee and hip operations which have nothing to do with their waistline. Fat children are bullied in schools; this has been going on for decades, but, sadly, the trend is on the increase. Anti-fat prejudice has become a global reality, and obesity has become associated with laziness and lack of self-control in almost every country of the world.

Maybe you grew up without a strong sense of *identity,* and being fat feels reassuring at some level, even though it makes you unhappy. Maybe it is a comfort zone that you're accustomed to, something stable in your life. Maybe you lack assertiveness, and your fat insulates you against others and the world in general. Like a protective layer, it gives you a ''thicker skin'. Overeating may help you cope with stress and with other people's behaviour. It can be a weapon against anger, frustration and despair. Once you lose weight you might become more sensitive, more aware of your feelings. You will need to handle them differently.

Fat may symbolize the lack of *control* you have over circumstances and people, the things you can't change. You can't force others to do things *your* way, or to stay with you. You can't force others to like you or to agree with you all the time. You can't expect them to feather your nest. Your happiness is no one's responsibility but your own. People may react differently to a skinny person, but it is up to you to *assert* yourself, in your family or in the workplace.

Your relationships will change dramatically once you let go of expectations and once you realize that you can't control others, but have the ability to make *yourself* happy.

Being your ideal weight won't take away your confidence. On the contrary, you will feel better within yourself, and generally more self-assured. You will look people in the eyes and smile at them more often, and the feedback you will receive is likely to be more favourable than when you were overweight. Maybe this frightens you, especially if you've been hiding behind your fat, which enabled you to create *space*, a kind of barrier to avoid closeness and intimacy. Maybe at some level you believe that you don't deserve this kind of interaction with people, or that you could set yourself up for hurt and disappointment.

Fear of abandonment goes back to early childhood and is deeply buried, ready to resurface when you're about to take the risk to be open and *vulnerable* in a relationship. Obesity makes you unavailable. It may also be a way to avoid a sexual relationship, as it can hamper your sex life.

Any positive emotion feels good and any negative emotion feels bad: comfort and discomfort/pleasure and pain. These basic emotions are eloquent in a newborn baby who cries when she's hungry, tired, lonely, too hot or too cold, frightened, has a dirty or wet nappy (diaper) or is in pain.

Pleasure, bliss, happiness, joy, satisfaction, relief, contentment and inner peace mean comfort. Pain, sadness, fear, anger, frustration and resentment mean discomfort. Due to upbringing and society's expectations, men are often more comfortable expressing anger, while women are more comfortable with sadness. Depression is becoming more common with both sexes though, and it is just another form of anger: anger turned inwards.

Listen to your 'gut feelings' and act accordingly, whenever it is appropriate and reasonable. If you feel good about a decision, then go ahead with it. If you feel uneasy about it, you're probably not meant to do it. However, it is beneficial to 'feel the fear and do it anyway'. If you don't get out of your comfort zone, you'll never do anything new or challenging. But you don't need to force yourself to do something if it doesn't feel right.

Timing is important, especially if you need to talk to someone about a difficult subject. Pay attention to your inner voice to make decisions that won't affect you or others in a negative way. If you're thinking about divorce, ask yourself how it will affect you as well as all other family members. You can pray to God, your Higher Power or the Universe for insight, guidance and support.

Maybe you eat when you're overwhelmed by negative emotions. When this happens, take a step back and look at the situation from a different perspective. Mindfulness can help you achieve this, by focusing your awareness on the present moment. You calmly acknowledge your thoughts, feelings and bodily sensations, without fighting them and without trying to escape from them. Bring your complete attention to the present moment, and accept it, without judging it and without trying to change it.

This very instant is the culmination of a long chain of events and decisions, made by *you* and by other people in the past. It doesn't just leap into existence without the events that have taken place prior to it. Usually, there are warning signs in life. For instance, when a relationship turns sour it normally doesn't happen overnight, but it is the result of months or years of miscommunication and mutual neglect.

Fear stems from the belief that you won't be able to cope with what lies ahead of you. But you have been able to cope with what's been happening so far. There is no reason why you should lose the ability to do this all of a sudden. You do have control over your future: you can determine your path. There is nothing to be afraid of. Fear of failure might paralyse you, but don't allow it to hold you back. Do everything it takes to lose weight, but don't focus on the outcome

Anger, an outward expression of hurt, fear and frustration, is not a bad thing in itself. This protective mechanism against a perceived loss of power can also be a positive energy that propels you forward. As a catalyst for change, anger may work like a trigger towards making a decision, and moving from a place where it hurts to a more favourable position. Anger can help you get out of a dissatisfying job or an abusive relationship. It can also help you lose weight, because you're furious at the way you've been overeating and neglecting yourself so far. This is *rightful* anger, not guilt.

When you're rightfully angry, you feel that something is not right; something needs to change. You can start by changing yourself, as you can't really change anyone else. You're responsible for your own happiness and self-worth. Don't give others the power to control your mind and your mood. Others might try to undermine or hurt you, but you're the one who agrees to take their pain on board and allows them to make you upset.

Feelings are an integral part of you and an important guidance system. Listen to them and analyse them as much as possible, but don't take action spontaneously as soon as you experience negative emotion; you could regret it later. When a bad feeling arises, don't do anything about it. Allow it to overcome you and observe the impact it has on you. It will subside eventually, like a wave that comes and goes. Emotions are just 'thoughts in motion', and it is their nature to be transitory. Sadness and grief often seem to last indefinitely, but their intensity will fade eventually.

An angry outburst can be fierce and frightening, but it's only a short-lived kind of madness. Feelings are not harmful, but the way you react to them can be. Emotions don't last forever, even though it often seems that way. To snap out of a negative emotion you could say to yourself, 'Let's see how long this will last.' As you practice this approach, you find that you remain upset for increasingly shorter periods of time.

Eating can be a way to repress or 'stuff down' painful emotions. 'Emotional eating' means you're using food to make yourself feel better, but emotional hunger can't be satisfied with food. Eating can alleviate bad feelings temporarily, but, as a coping mechanism, it doesn't work, because the problem is still there. Your expanding waistline and feelings of guilt and shame about overeating aggravate the situation. Consequently, you don't attempt to deal with issues in a healthier way, and your weight spirals out of control. It's a vicious circle, as you now feel more and more powerless over both food *and* your emotions.

In the masterpiece of French literature *The Little Prince*, by Antoine de Saint-Exupery, the little prince asks a drunkard *why* he drinks. The drunkard replies that he does it because he wants to forget. When the Little Prince enquires *what* he wants to forget, the drunkard answers, 'To forget that I'm ashamed.' 'Ashamed of what?' asks the little prince. 'Ashamed of drinking!' says the drunkard.

Mood fluctuations compound the problem of having to deal with painful emotions. If you suffer from mood swings, a diet high in complex carbohydrates can help you remain calm and in control. It will enhance serotonin production in your brain and alleviate restlessness, anxiety and depression. SSRI (Selective Serotonin Reuptake Inhibitor) antidepressants do the same thing: they increase serotonin levels, promoting feelings of wellbeing rather than discomfort. To include complex carbs in your diet can make a huge difference to your state of mind and how you feel throughout the day.

Eating less and moving more may well be the keys to dropping extra kilograms, but there is much more to the weight loss equation. It's good to know the theory, but it's not enough: you need to be able to put it into practice and stick with it. It seems to work well when things are running smoothly, but a soon as something adverse happens, you get upset and you reach for food. When you're stressed, you eat to stop yourself from feeling bad: food is your safety valve. The secret is to look for comfort and support in other areas of your life. Nurture yourself in ways that don't involve food. Eating may be the only thing you enjoy. But if you put a little thought into it, you can find other techniques to enhance your life, lighten your burdens and grant yourself some leisure time.

Key Points and Strategies:

- Find out what being *heavy* means to you: not just on the surface, but also underneath
- Ask yourself what you're afraid of and what makes you angry
- Use the positive energy of anger to motivate you to lose weight in a *healthy* way
- Completely accept the present moment and your emotions without judgment
- Listen to your inner voice, your guidance system, instead of suppressing it
- Acknowledge your negative feelings, and practice mindfulness to defuse them
- Don't reach for food when you feel low. Adopt new coping mechanisms
- Don't 'stuff your feelings' with emotional eating

- Find out what makes you feel better and what helps you relax
- Look after yourself and nurture yourself, so you won't have the urge to overeat.

CONCLUSION

Don't dwell on the past. Don't worry about the future. Focus on the present moment, and eliminate the word 'failure' from your vocabulary.

The reason why I became a nutrition, diet and weight loss expert is partly due to my background as a Registered Nurse and Counsellor, as well as my personal experience. A mother of six children and a proud grandmother, I was pregnant six times. Each time, I gained a tremendous amount of weight: twenty 20 kilograms for each pregnancy on average! Every time, I managed to lose this excess weight (120 kilograms altogether) over a period of one or two years following my pregnancies. Today I weigh the same as I did thirty years ago. How did I manage to avoid left over baby weight as well as middle age spread? By adhering to the principles in this book, which are simple, straightforward and easy to understand!

It was a long journey, which started about two decades ago, when I had trouble losing weight after my second pregnancy. Two years after the birth of my second son, I was still carrying a lot of excess weight. I felt bloated, unfit and tired most of the time. None of my pre-pregnancy clothes fit me, and I didn't want to go shopping, for fear I would have to buy plus size clothes! I felt miserable and my self-esteem was in the toilet. I had never been model skinny, but my weight had always been in the normal range for my height. After my second baby, I felt like a big fat blob! This made me angry, and I was ready to change!

I didn't quite know how to go about the whole weight loss thing. I despised the word 'diet': that four letter word made me cringe. I wasn't willing to starve or deprive myself, so I had to find an alternative to the traditional, draconian way of dieting. I was looking for a pain-free weight loss method that *worked*. Besides looking good, I wanted to feel good and have perfect health. I was looking for strategies to lose and maintain a normal or ideal weight, as well as promoting optimum health and longevity – guaranteed way to shed kilograms permanently, without the risk of rebound weight gain once the diet was over.

A diet is never over. It is not something you do for a few weeks or months, then give up and revert to unhealthy eating habits. It's a way of life. The method I devised is easy to follow. You can do it for the rest of your life, while experiencing the magic of being transformed, body and mind. It's not a daunting chore, but an exciting adventure and a path of pure enjoyment, once a few obstacles and misconceptions have been removed. I wanted to clear away diet myths and reveal the real truth, based on science, about successful weight loss and healthy eating. It's all about adopting good habits based on sound strategies and biological principles.

Once new habits take root, they become *automatic*. They require less and less willpower as they become an integral part of you, a natural aspect of your daily routine. Willpower may only be necessary in the beginning. The more motivated you are, the easier it will be for you to stick to your resolutions. To fuel your desire and your determination, look forward to the end result, and seek joy in the entire journey, the process. By visualizing what you want to achieve, while cultivating positive thoughts and enthusiasm, you'll stay on the right track. You won't stray and you will arrive at your destination. Be patient and trust yourself and your abilities.

I researched weight loss for two decades. Besides reading every diet book I could put my hands on, I talked to people who had lost weight successfully and maintained their newfound shape. I wanted to find out what worked for them. Whenever something made sense and resonated with me, I wrote it down, until finally, I held a manuscript in my hands. I put it aside for almost twenty years, and only recently dug it out. I revised it completely in the light of new research and new science discoveries. For instance, in the nineties, we thought that fat was responsible for making us overweight or obese. But this myth has been debunked, and today it is a consensus that fat is actually good for you and even *necessary*, in moderation and as long as it's the right kind of fat.

To reach your goal, understand and improve your relationship with food, exercise and your body. Analyse yourself and find out where you went wrong in the past. But don't dwell on your mistakes; put them behind and turn over a new leaf. Don't dream too much of the future either. Instead, concentrate on the present moment. Your maximum point of power is NOW.

☼ **In brief:**

- Make healthy food choices today, with a focus on plant-based foods
- Get the right fuel: wholesome nutrition, no junk food
- Stay away from processed foods
- Avoid the sugar trap
- Avoid cooking and frying in fat
- Eliminate trans fats
- Increase your consumption of fresh fruit and vegetables
- Eat legumes, seeds and nuts
- Think complex carbs and fibre (e.g. whole grains, brown rice, vegetables, beans)
- Include super foods in your diet
- Keep alcohol to a minimum

- Drink plenty of water
- Do some moderate-intensity physical activity.

There is no such thing as failure. You can pick yourself up, analyse what went wrong, learn the lessons and start again. Use the present moment and live in it consciously, to the fullest. The more you seek fulfilment *now* and enjoy your body *as it is*, the more you'll be likely to achieve your weight loss goal and maintain your new body shape. If you're critical and judgmental of yourself now, you will remain that way, no matter how many clothes sizes you drop.

You can only lose weight if it is what you *really* want. Believe that you *deserve* to be your ideal shape. Prepare yourself and start caring for yourself *now*. Put yourself first and take yourself seriously. Don't wait to lose weight to feel grateful and appreciate yourself as the miracle of creation that you are.

Self-acceptance and awareness, as well as loving yourself are the top ingredients of your recipe for success.

With all my love and warmest wishes,

Bella Tindale
Forest Lakes, October 30, 2014.

APPENDIX

Difference between Type 1 and Type 2 Diabetes.

Australians are getting heavier and the average young Australian has gained a whopping 6.7 kg since the year 2000. Diabetes is soon to become the number one cause of death and illness in Australia, where presently 1.5 million people live with the disease. It is estimated that by 2025, 3 million people will be affected. Sensible dieting will prevent Diabetes, your number one health risk.

There are two types of Diabetes:

- **Type 1:** The body is producing NO insulin. This person needs regular insulin injections for the rest of their life.
- **Type 2:** Insulin is *present* but in insufficient amount; or the cells don't respond correctly to insulin. Oral medication may be necessary to lower their blood sugar levels. Insulin injections are required if oral tablets alone can't control blood sugar levels. Sometimes it is possible to control diabetes type 2 by diet and exercise alone, especially in the early stages.

Type 1 Diabetes is an *autoimmune* disease: the person's own body has destroyed the insulin-producing cells in the pancreas. This type of diabetes is also known as Juvenile Diabetes or Childhood Diabetes, as it is extremely rare for it to appear after the age of 40. People with Type 1 have to inject insulin regularly in order to stay alive. This type of diabetes is *not* preventable. There is a genetic predisposition for it, while the environmental risk factors are still unclear. The presence of certain antibodies (which may be triggered by a virus) in the blood may be a precursor of the disease.

In Type 2 Diabetes, there is not enough insulin produced, or the insulin is not working properly (this is called insulin *resistance*). 85 % of people affected by the disease have Type 2, which is totally preventable, as it depends on diet and lifestyle. Genetics play an important role, but so does lifestyle. Studies have shown that you can delay or prevent type 2 Diabetes by exercising and losing weight. The vast majority of people develop the condition because they are overweight or unfit. This type of diabetes tends to appear later in life, but there are more and more cases of people in their twenties with the disease, and even in children as young as twelve year olds.

Type 2 diabetes is prevalent in Australia today because we have all the contributing factors: sedentary lifestyle, easy access to processed food, weight gain and a multicultural society with people from high-risk genetic backgrounds, such as Indigenous, Chinese, Indian, Africans and Pacific Islanders. The long-term implications of diabetes are scary: blindness, amputation, kidney failure and heart attack. And yet may people seem to ignore the alarm bells, with rates of the disease soaring across the globe. People are eating more and more 'empty' calories, foods that are high in energy: high in sugar, fat and salt, but low in essential nutrients, vitamins and fibre.

The food industry spends billions of dollars every year to develop new products, attractive packaging, as well as powerful advertising and marketing techniques to entice us to purchase more food. Selling more food means more profit for these companies. Through advertising and the media, we are constantly encouraged to buy products we don't need, and this includes food such as soft drinks (soda), fries and burgers.

Popular fast food chains have been blamed for the obesity epidemic, and for directly targeting young children, but they are not solely responsible. Supermarket shelves are stacked to the brim with a wide variety of chocolate bars, cookies, cakes, pastries, crackers, biscuits, lollies (candy) and chips (crisps). There are rows of sugary cereals and huge freezers with every possible variety and flavour of ice-cream. Processed food is often cheaper than fresh food, and it is often cheaper to eat fast food than to buy the ingredients for a nutritious meal at home.

Being overweight or obese is the single most important thing that predicts who will develop Type 2 Diabetes. Following this book's suggestions will put you on the right path to prevent this debilitating condition. Type 2 Diabetes is a chronic disease that can have serious, negative impacts on your entire body. As well as affecting your health and wellbeing, it may considerably shorten your lifespan. Losing extra weight, eating health and becoming physically more active are the three most important things you can do to remain diabetes-free.

Moderate exercise and diabetes

For people with diabetes, physical activity improves the body's response to *insulin*, which lowers blood sugar levels. Less medication or insulin injections may be needed as a result. Exercise also reduces the risk of developing long-term diabetes complications which affect the eyes, feet, kidneys, heart and blood vessels. Over a period of time, high blood glucose levels damage the small and large blood vessels and nerves. Exercise offers protection, especially together with a healthy diet, as it lowers blood glucose, and keeps blood vessels and nerves in good shape.

FURTHER READING

Bilderback, Leslie and Nissenberg, Sandra K., M.S., R.D. *The Everything Family Nutrition Book: All You Need to Keep Your Family Healthy, Active and Strong.* Avon, Massachusetts: Adams Media, 2009.

Blatner, Dawn, Jackson, R.D., L.D.N. *The Flexitarian Diet: The Mostly Vegetarian Way to Lose Weight, Be Healthier, Prevent Disease, and Add Years to Your life. 140 Quick and Delicious Recipes.* New York: McGraw-Hill Books, 2010.

Brand-Miller, Jennie, Dr. *The Low GI Diet Revolution: The Definite Science-Based Weight Loss Plan.* New York: Marlowe & Company, 2005. This book was first published in Australia in 2004 under the title *The Low GI Diet* by Hodder Headline Australia.

Brazier, Brendan. *Thrive Foods: 200 Plant-Based Recipes for Peak Health.* Toronto, Ontario: Penguin Group (Canada), 2011.

Burrell, Susie. *Losing the Last Five Kilos. Simple Steps to Get the Body You Want Now.* London: Hardie Grant Books, 2010.

Bussell, Jason, MSOM, Licensed Acupuncturist. *The Asian Diet. Simple Secrets for Eating Right, Losing Weight and Being Well.* Forres, Scotland: Findhorn Press, 2009.

Cabot, Sandra, Dr. *The Liver Cleansing Diet. Love Your Liver and Live Longer!* Paddington, New South Wales, Australia: Women's Health Advisory Service, 1996.

Chopra, Deepak, M.D. *What Are You Hungry For? The Chopra Solution to Permanent Weight Loss, Well-Being, and Lightness of Soul.* New York: Harmony Books, 2013.

CSIRO (Commonwealth Scientific and Industrial Research Organisation). *The CSIRO Total Wellbeing Diet. Recipes on a Budget.* Melbourne: Viking Australia, 2013.

CSIRO and BAKER IDI (International Diabetes Institute). *The CSIRO Diabetes and Lifestyle Plan.* Collingwood, Victoria: CSIRO Publishing, 2011.

Dean, Carolyn, M.D., N.D. *The Magnesium Miracle. Discover the missing link to total health: Lower the risk of heart disease. Prevent stroke and obesity. Treat diabetes. Improve mood and memory.* New York: Ballantine Books, 2003.

Doyle, William and Moriyama, Naomi. *The Japan Diet: The Secret to Effective and Lasting Weight Loss.* London: Vermilion, 2007.

Dunne, Carolyn. *The Semi-Vegetarian Cookbook: Simple to Prepare Gourmet Recipes for a Healthy Lifestyle.* New York: Bantam Books, 1989.

Gayler, Paul and Heiser, Gemma. *Healthy Eating for Lower Blood Pressure: 100 Delicious Recipes from an Expert Team of Chef and Nutritionist.* London: Kyle Books, 2011.

Good Housekeeping Institute. Easy to Make! Low GI. Over 100 Triple-Tested Recipes. London: Collins & Brown, 2011.

Harrison, John, Dr. *Love your Disease: It's Keeping You Healthy.* Sydney: HarperCollins Publishers Australia, 1986.

Itsiopoulos, Catherine, Dr. *The Mediterranean Diet*. Australia: Pan Macmillan, 2013.

Lustig, Robert H., M.D. *Fat Chance. Beating the Odds Against Sugar, Processed Food, Obesity and Disease*. New York: Hudson Street Press, 2013.

Madison, Deborah. *Vegetable Literacy: Cooking and Gardening with Twelve Families from the Edible Plant Kingdom, with over 300 Deliciously Simple Recipes*. Berkeley, California: Ten Speed Press, 2013.

May, Michelle, M.D. *Eat What You Love, Love What You Eat: How to Break Your Eat-Repent-Repeat Cycle*. Austin, Texas: Greenleaf Book Group.

Meyer, Joyce. *Eat and Stay Thin. Simple, Spiritual, Satisfying Weight Control*. Fenton, Missouri: Life in the Word, Warner Books Edition, 2002.

Matheny, Sarah. *Peas and Thank You. Simple Meatless Meals the Whole Family will Love*. Don Mills, Ontario, Canada: Harlequin, 2011.

Mindell's, Earl, RPh., PhD. *Soy Miracle: How adding soy foods to your diet may protect you against diseases such as prostate and breast cancer, osteoporosis, and coronary artery disease*. New York: Fireside, Simon & Schuster, 1995.

Moore, Michael. *Blood Sugar: Inspiring Recipes for Anyone Facing the Challenges of Diabetes and Maintaining Good Health*. Australia: New Holland, 2011.

Moss, Michael. *Salt, Sugar Fat: How the Food Giants Hooked Us*. New York: Random House, 2013.

Noakes, Manny, Dr. with Clifton, Peter, Dr. *The CSIRO Total Wellbeing Diet.* Melbourne: Penguin Books Australia, 2005.

Orbach, Susan. *Fat is a Feminine Issue.* London: Arrow Books Random House, 1998.

Patel, Raj R., M.D. *The Healthy Indian Diet. How Traditional Foods of South Asia Help Prevent Heart Disease, Diabetes and Cancer.* Sun Health Press at Create Space, 2011.

Podleski, Janet and Podleski, Greta. *The Looneyspoons Collection: Good Food, Good Health, Good Fun!* Carlsbad, California: Hay House, 2012.

Roth, Geneen. *Feeding the Hungry Heart. The Experience of Compulsive Eating.* Indianapolis, Indiana: Bobbs-Merrill, 1982

Schaef, Anne Wilson. *When Society Becomes an Addict.* Harper, San Francisco, 1987.

Simon, Julie M. *The Emotional Eater's Repair Manual. A Practical Mind-Body-Spirit Guide for Putting an End to Overeating and Dieting.* Novato, California: New World Library, 2012.

Spencer, Stan, PhD. *The Diet's Dropout Guide to Natural Weight Loss: Find Your Easiest Path to Naturally Thin.* Riverside, California: Fine Life Books, 2013.

Stone, Gene (Editor), Campbell, Colin T., PhD and Esselstyn, Caldwell B., Jr., MD. *Forks Over Knives: The Plant-Based Way to Health.* New York: The Experiment, 2011.

Straten, Michael van. *The Complete Superfoods Cookbook: Dishes and Drinks for Energy, Detoxing and Health.* London: Octopus Publishing Group, 2007.

Williamson, Marianne. *A Course in Weight Loss. 21 Spiritual Lessons for Surrendering Your Weight Forever.* Carlsbad, California: Hay House, 2010.

Wurtman, Judith J., PhD. *The Serotonin Solution.* New York: Ballantine Books, 1996.

Zuckerbrot, Tanya, MS, RD. *The Miracle Carb Diet: Make Calories and Fat Disappear–with Fiber!* New York: HarperCollins, 2012.